PEDIATRIC
NURSING
SECRETS

PEDIATRIC NURSING SECRETS

SUZANNE M. LEVASSEUR, MSN, APRN, CPNP
Pediatric Nurse Practitioner
Broadview Middle School
School Based Health Center
Danbury, Connecticut

HANLEY & BELFUS, INC. / Philadelphia

Publisher: HANLEY & BELFUS, INC.
                  Medical Publishers
                  210 South 13th Street
                  Philadelphia, PA 19107
                  (215) 546-7293; 800-962-1892
                  FAX (215) 790-9330
                  Web site: http://www.hanleyandbelfus.com

Note to the reader: Although the information in this book has been carefully reviewed for correctness of dosage and indications, neither the authors nor the editor nor the publisher can accept any legal responsibility for any errors or omissions that may be made. Neither the publisher nor the editor makes any warranty, expressed or implied, with respect to the material contained herein. Before prescribing any drug, the reader must review the manufacturer's current product information (package inserts) for accepted indications, absolute dosage recommendations, and other information pertinent to the safe and effective use of the product described.

Library of Congress Control Number: 2002102756

PEDIATRIC NURSING SECRETS   ISBN 1-56053-522-9

Last digit is the print number: 9 8 7 6 5 4 3 2 1

CONTENTS

CONTRIBUTORS

Deborah Bibeau, RN, MSN
Arrhythmia Case Manager, Division of Pediatric Cardiology, Vanderbilt University Medical Center, Nashville, Tennessee

Joseann Helmes DeWitt, RN, MSN, C, CLNC
Assistant Professor, Department of Baccalaureate Nursing, Alcorn State University School of Nursing, Natchez, Mississippi

Elaine M. Gustafson, MSN, APRN, CS, PNP
Assistant Professor, Department of Pediatric Nurse Practitioner Specialty, Yale University School of Nursing; Fair Haven Community Health Center, New Haven, Connecticut

Beth F. Hallmark, RN, MSN
Instructor and Course Coordinator, Department of Child and Family Nursing, Belmont University School of Nursing, Nashville, Tennessee

Andrea M. Kline, RN, MS, CCRN, PCCNP
Pediatric Critical Care Nurse Practitioner, Pediatric Intensive Care Unit, Children's Memorial Hospital, Chicago, Illinois

Suzanne M. Levasseur, MSN, APRN, CPNP
Pediatric Nurse Practitioner, Broadview Middle School, School Based Health Center, Danbury, Connecticut

Kathleen M. Moonan, RNC, MS, IBCLC
Lactation Consultant, Danbury Hospital, Danbury, Connecticut

Patricia Morel Murphy, RNC, MSN, IBCLC
Lactation Coordinator, Danbury Hospital, Danbury, Connecticut

Diana Odland Neal, RN, MS
Assistant Professor of Nursing, St. Olaf College, Northfield, Minnesota

Delia R. Nickolaus, RN, MSN
Clinical Nurse Educator, Vanderbilt Children's Hospital, Nashville, Tennessee

Linda J. Allan Pasto, MS, RN
Professor, Department of Nursing, Tompkins-Cortland Community College, Dryden, New York

Patricia Ryan-Krause, MS, RN, MSN, APRN
Assistant Professor, Department of Pediatrics, Yale University School of Nursing, New Haven, Connecticut; Pediatric Nurse Practitioner, Children's Medical Group, Hamden, Connecticut

Barbara Hoyer Schaffner, PhD, RN, CPNP
Professor of Nursing, Otterbein College, Westerville, Ohio

Rebecca L. Shabo, RN, CPNP, PhD
Associate Professor of Nursing, Georgia Baptist College of Nursing of Mercer University, Atlanta, Georgia

Lauren R. Sorce, RN, MSN, CCRN, CPNP
Pediatric Nurse Practitioner, Pediatric Critical Care Unit, Children's Memorial Hospital, Chicago, Illinois

Joyce Weishaar, RN, MSN, CCNS
Clinical Nurse Specialist, Pediatric Intensive Care Unit, Children's Memorial Hospital, Chicago, Illinois

Bruce K. Wilson, PhD
Associate Professor, Nursing Department, University of Texas–Pan American College of Health Sciences and Human Services, Edinburg, Texas

Karen Wolownik, RNC, MSN, CPNP
Pediatric Blood and Marrow Transplant Coordinator, Department of Pediatric Oncology, Children's Hospital of New York-Presbyterian, University Hospitals of Columbia and Cornell, New York, New York

PREFACE

Nurses who care for children and their families have a love and passion for the work they do and are in continued pursuit of knowledge and skills to provide better care for their patients. Everyone in the specialty of pediatric nursing knows that children are not just small adults but have a unique set of physical, psychological, and emotional needs. The nurse who works with the pediatric patient must have an extensive knowledge base about pediatric growth and development, pediatric disease processes, the emotional needs of the hospitalized child, and the ever-challenging aspect of working with families of ill children.

This book is designed to provide an interesting and fun way to obtain valuable information about caring for the child from infancy through adolescence. It covers the realm of well-child and school-based care through the highly complex care of the critically ill child. The format of questions and answers presents the information in a concise, easy, and enjoyable way. Although not meant to be a comprehensive text covering all pediatric nursing concepts, this text is nonetheless a valuable asset to all nurses who work exclusively with children as well as to nurses in other specialties who occasionally care for children, including emergency department, recovery room, and outpatient office nurses. The many "secrets" and pearls of wisdom in this book will enhance nursing care and positively impact pediatric patients and their families.

Suzanne M. Levasseur, MSN, APRN, CPNP

ACKNOWLEDGMENTS

I would like to acknowledge and thank all the chapter authors, who come from diverse professional settings, for their expertise and commitment to this project. A special thanks goes to Linda Scheetz, the Nursing Secrets Series® editor, for involving me in this project and for her tireless patience, guidance, and eye for detail. My gratitude also goes out to all my interdisciplinary colleagues who work with children everyday with dedication, compassion, and enthusiasm.

1. CHILD DEVELOPMENT

Elaine M. Gustafson, MSN, APRN, CS, PNP

CLINICAL ISSUES

1. How many parents raise concerns about child development when they bring their child for well-child care?

One quarter to one third.

2. What percentage of children in the United States have developmental or behavioral disabilities?

Approximately 15–18%.

3. What percentage of children experience school failure or drop out of high school?

7–10%.

4. Do parents have adequate time with the clinician to address their concerns?

Apparently not. According to one U.S. study, patients are allowed to speak for 18 seconds before being interrupted by the physician, and when interrupted, only 2% finish their statement or question.

5. List the goals of relationship-based health care practice.

- Build relationships to provide services to children and families
- Recognize that the relationship between the parent and practitioner is fundamental to quality service
- Promote the parent–child relationship

6. List the hallmarks of relationship-based practice.

- Set an agenda in collaboration with the parents to highlight parents' strengths and expertise
- Encourage parents to consider the child's perception of events
- Convey an atmosphere of reciprocity between parent and child

7. Describe some basic principles of growth and development.

1. Development is **complex**. It is continuous, irreversible, and lifelong.
2. Development has **direction**. It follows a sequence.
3. Development is **predictable**. It may occur early or late.

8. List some of the multiple interactive forces that may influence child development.

Culture and lifestyle	*Physical environment*
Cultural input	Intrauterine conditions
Gender socialization	Home environment
Family structure	School environment
Single-parent families, blended families	*Socioeconomic status*
Styles of parenting	Poverty
	Lack of parental education
	High unemployment
	Residential crowding

PSYCHOSOCIAL ISSUES

9. Define *intellectual competency*.

A composite of skills, behaviors, and adaptive abilities that make it possible for an individual to adapt to new situations, to think abstractly, and to profit from experiences.

10. What is the basis of Piaget's theory of cognitive development?

Assimilation and **accommodation**; that is, living organisms interact with the environment by changing it and changing themselves. This theory presupposes active participation in the process of learning. Children learn from the external world by actively interacting with it.

11. Name the four stages of development attributed to Piaget and the corresponding ages for each stage.

    1. Sensorimotor period: 0–2 years
    2. Preoperational period: 2–7 years
    3. Concrete operational period: 7–11 years
    4. Formal operational period: >11 years

12. What developmental hallmarks characterize each of Piaget's stages?

STAGE	HALLMARKS
Sensorimotor period	**Object permanence**—Child is unable to separate self from objects in the environment. Child has limited ability to anticipate consequences of actions.
Preoperational period	**Egocentricism**—Child is unable to distinguish easily between his own perspective and that of someone else. **Animism**—Child believes that inanimate objects have human qualities and are capable of human action.
Concrete operational period	**Relativism**—Child is able to operate with two or more aspects of a problem (e.g., able to relate to both time and space). **Reversibility**—Child is able to mentally reverse actions (e.g., perform arithmetic problems, mentally pour liquids back and forth).
Formal operational period	**Hypothetical reasoning**—Ability to function on a symbolic abstract level, capable of deductive hypothesis testing.

13. Describe the components of the personality structures inherent in Freud's psychoanalytic theory.

- **Id** is the unconscious source of motives and drives (i.e., pleasure principle or need for immediate gratification).
- **Ego** represents logic and reason and mediates between id, superego, and reality.
- **Superego** incorporates moral values and standards into personality and modifies id impulses.

14. Explain the Oedipus complex and its implications.

According to Freud, the Oedipus complex is the love attachment of a preschool child to the parent of the opposite sex and a wish to get rid of the same-sex parent. It is not considered to be a central developmental process today but rather a normal phase of development during which these conflicts are resolved and seldom remembered.

15. Describe the characteristics of Erikson's theory of psychosocial development.

Erikson's theory stresses the importance of social factors. It is characterized by psychosocial crises represented by a conflict between an individual and society. The resolution of each crisis enhances the ability of the individual to resolve the next crisis. This process continues throughout the life span.

16. List the stages of psychosocial development as described by Erikson, the inherent conflict, and the expected outcome.

STAGE	CONFLICT	OUTCOME
0–18 mo	Trust vs. mistrust	Trust
18 mo	Autonomy vs. shame	Feeling of adequacy
Preschool	Initiative vs. guilt	Purposefulness
6–11 yr	Industry vs. inferiority	Competence
Adolescent	Identity vs. role confusion	Self-identity

17. What are the levels of attachment as described in Bowlby's attachment theory?

0–3 months Undiscriminating social responsiveness characterized by visual fixation, grasping, smiling, and crying

3–6 months Discriminating social responsiveness in which the child distinguishes between family and nonfamily (mother vs. stranger)

6–24 months Active initiative in which the child actively engages in relationships by following and greeting others

18. Name two other attachment processes in the young child.

1. **Stranger anxiety** (approximately 8 months): Child may exhibit a fearful responses to strangers.

2. **Separation anxiety** (approximately 1 year): Child displays a fearful response when left by caretaker.

19. What are the functions of attachment?
- Provide a sense of security
- Regulate affect and arousal
- Promote the expression of feelings and communication
- Serve as a basis for exploration

20. List some typical responses of children subjected to prolonged separation from parents as a result of hospitalization.
- **Protest**—crying, screaming, physical resistance (e.g., kicking)
- **Despair**—withdrawal, feeling hopeless
- **Detachment**—recovers from misery, accepts attention from others, may react with disinterest when parents visit

21. Name the levels of childhood temperament and some possible characteristics of and responses to each level.

Difficult child
Responds best to scheduled feedings and structured caregiving
Functions well when knows the rules
Not dependent on people—natural leader
Competitive—seeks activity during stress

Easy child
Adapts readily to any situation
May sleep for prolonged intervals, may need to be awakened to feed
Friendly, smiles, laughs
Sleeps and eats well
Seeks people during stress

Slow to warm-up child
Socially shy
Avid reader
Poor relaxer
Highly distractible child
Requires additional soothing measures
Responds to swinging, being carried in pack
High-activity child
Requires vigilant watching
Requires extra safety measure in the home
Benefits from gross motor activities to channel energy

22. What does *goodness of fit* mean in parent-child relationships?
This refers to the parent's understanding of the child's temperament. Based on this understanding, parents clarify their expectations, aspirations, and caregiving style.

LANGUAGE DEVELOPMENT

23. Describe three theories of language development.
1. **Innate theory** assumes that acquisition of language is genetically determined.
2. **Reinforcement theory** proposes that language is learned as a result of environmental interactions.
3. **Social learning theory** proposes that language is acquired as a result of a modeling process resulting from imitation of adult remarks and reinforcement by adults.

24. What are some implications of language development for parents and health care providers?
- Because **receptive (comprehensive) language** occurs first, clinicians may encourage parents to talk frequently to their infants. Clinicians can model this behavior before, during, and after care.
- As children develop **expressive language**, praise is important because approval results in more effective language skills.

DEVELOPMENTAL MEASURES AND MILESTONES

25. List the domains of development that are assessed in the Denver Developmental Screening Test (DDST).
- Personal and social skills
- Gross motor skills
- Language skills
- Fine motor skills

26. What is the targeted age range for the DDST?
Newborn to age 6.

27. What developmental milestones can be observed in the first weeks of life?
Newborns will begin to:
- Follow objects with their eyes
- Look at faces
- Respond to sounds by startling, blinking, crying, or quieting

28. What question may help a clinician gain some important insights into the future hopes of new parents for their infant?
"How did you choose your child's name? Does the name have some special significance for you?"

29. Define *mutual regulation*.

A process by which a parent or caregiver supports a child's attempt at self-regulation by providing structure and routine and by responsive interactions.

30. Why is mutual regulation important to infants and toddlers?

Without self-regulation, infants become fussy and disorganized with consequent disruption of family routines that can result in chaos.

31. How can parents support their child's efforts at self-regulation?

Parents need to learn to read and respond to their child's cues; this creates an interactive dynamic, beneficial to the infant and the parent. Parents need to be aware that learning self-regulation is a necessary child developmental task that their infant/toddler must master.

32. Define middle childhood.

Middle childhood is the period between pre-school years and adolescence—the elementary school years. This period is characterized by a sense of industry and accomplishment.

33. What physical changes can be expected in middle childhood?

The child experiences a slower growth rate than in previous years but does develop major increases in strength and coordination. This contributes to the child's growing sense of competence in relation to physical abilities and supports efforts at participation in sports and other physical pursuits.

34. List some achievements of middle childhood.
- Responsibility for good health habits
- Belief in capacity for success
- Awareness of rules of safety
- Ability to read, write, and communicate increasingly complex and creative thoughts
- Identification with peer group
- Responsibility for homework and school achievement

35. List some tasks for the school-age child.
- Practice good dental hygiene
- Maintain good eating habits and appropriate weight
- Resist peer pressure to engage in risk-taking behaviors
- Control impulses, resolve conflict, and manage anger
- Assume responsibility for belongings, chores, and good health habits
- Communicate well with parents, teachers, and other adults
- Be industrious in school

PARENTAL INFLUENCES

36. How can parents enhance the development of their school-age child?
1. Show interest in the child's school performance and after-school activities.
2. Encourage self-responsibility.
3. Show affection in the family.
4. Know the child's friends and their families.
5. Share meals as a family whenever possible.
6. Encourage good sibling relationships, attempt to resolve conflicts without taking sides, and do not allow violence.
7. Participate in games and physical activity with the child.

37. List some effects of prolonged television watching.
- Increase in aggressive behavior
- Difficulty distinguishing fantasy from reality
- Distorted perceptions of reality
- Trivialization of sex and sexuality

38. What counseling should health care providers give to parents regarding television watching?

The American Academy of Pediatrics recommends the following:
- Set limits on amount of television a child watches. Parents should decide how early they want to start their child watching television.
- Help the child plan television viewing in advance, remembering that homework comes first.
- Do not allow television watching during dinner.
- Do not allow a child to have a television in his or her bedroom.
- Set an example of the behavior you wish to instill in your child (e.g., reading, exercise).
- Visit the library often with your child.

39. Define "ghosts in the nursery" and describe their implications.

Fraiberg used the phrase "ghosts in the nursery" to describe "visitors from parents' unremembered past," or unresolved psychological issues or dysfunctional family dynamics from the parents' childhood that influence how the parents interact with their own child. These ghosts can contribute significantly to the child's personality development and to the parent–child relationship.

40. List some ghosts in the nursery.
- Insecure attachment of parents to own parents
- Parents with detachment difficulties from overly controlling parents
- Parents hoped for a child of a different gender
- A deceased child or grandparent whom the child replaced

41. What approach may help clinicians address difficult topics, such as domestic violence, depression, substance abuse, and guns, with parents?

Frame such questions with: "It is my job to help you to be the best parent that you can be, so I need to ask you about...."

42. List concerns that may arise in children of depressed mothers.
- Significant behavioral difficulties
- Self-control issues
- Poor peer relationships
- Academic difficulties, including attention problems
- Risk for affective disorders

43. List some characteristics of resilience in children.
- Ability to function competently under threat or to recover from extreme stress or trauma quickly
- Capacity to meet a challenge and use it for psychological growth
- Achievement of good developmental outcomes and adaptive abilities despite growing up in high-risk situations

44. List protective factors that are associated with a resilient child.
Good health
Good-natured temperament
Above-average intelligence

Positive self-esteem
Active response to stress
Ability to seek help appropriately

45. What parental characteristics enhance resilience in a child?
- Secure attachment
- Parental warmth
- Good caregiving after stressful experience
- Modeling of coping skills and competent behavior
- Rules and structure in home
- Monitoring of child's behavior

46. List the fundamental goals of discipline.
To teach children to:
- Understand the effects of their behavior on others
- Respect the needs of others
- Weigh self-needs with needs of others
- Make choices based on self-needs and needs of others

47. What do children need to behave appropriately?
- Clear expectations
- Predictability
- Balance of power
- Acknowledgment of feelings
- Experience of the consequences of their choices

ADOLESCENCE

48. What are the three psychosocial developmental phases of adolescence?
1. Early (11–14 years): middle school
2. Middle (15–17 years): high school
3. Late (18–21 years)

49. List the three domains of growth in adolescence with the characteristics of each.
1. **Physical:** Increased height and weight, onset of menarche or spermarche, development of secondary sex characteristics
2. **Cognitive:** Increased cognitive capacity, change in thinking from concrete to abstract
3. **Emotional:** Increased intimacy with peers, decreased time with family, increased importance of peer group

50. Describe some general principles that govern the process of psychosocial development and help define the range of normal behavior in adolescence.
- Thinking ability moves from concrete to **abstract thought**, allowing adolescents to translate experiences into abstract ideas and to think about the consequences of their actions.
- **Everyday issues**, such as school, clothing, hairstyles, and chores, are the usual sources of conflict in the family. Disruptive family conflict is not the norm.
- **Transition** into adulthood is usually continuous and smooth. It is not usually a time of storm and stress.

51. In what ways is egocentrism played out in adolescence?
Imaginary audience. Adolescents often are obsessed with bodily changes brought about by puberty. These changes coupled with the ability to think abstractly create the notion that everyone is thinking about and noticing them.

Personal fable. Adolescents often believe that "if everyone is thinking about and watching me, then I must be special" and the laws of nature do not apply to them. This belief explains risk-taking behavior of adolescence and the "it can't happen to me attitude."

Overthinking. Adolescents often make things much more complicated than they are and read things into situations that are not there. For example, an adolescent may assume that a teacher hates him or her because he or she was not called on in class.

Apparent hypocrisy. Adolescents often have the notion that rules apply differently to them than they do to others. An adolescent may think that he or she should have free access to a parent's car, while believing that the parent does not need to know when or where he or she is going.

52. Describe the three types of adolescent autonomy.

1. **Emotional:** Adolescents develop close relationships and begin to weigh personal priorities (e.g., spending time with a boyfriend or girlfriend vs. hanging out with friends).

2. **Behavioral:** Adolescents make independent decisions and carry them out. They often seek advice from friends about social issues, from teachers and other adults for objective information, and from parents about values and future plans.

3. **Values:** Adolescents develop a set of principles about right and wrong. They may challenge family and societal values in the process.

53. At what age do parental conflicts peak?

15–17 years (during middle adolescence).

54. What types of issues may lead to parental conflicts?

Adolescents may argue and renegotiate issues of independence, such as curfews, dating, and driving.

55. Why is the development of adolescent autonomy a challenge for families?

Autonomy is a necessary part of adolescent development and is essential to the transition to adulthood. The challenge is for families to provide adolescents with the opportunity to test limits and boundaries within a safe environment.

BIBLIOGRAPHY

1. Betz CL, Hunsberger M, Wright S, Foster RLR: Family-Centered Nursing Care of Children, 2nd ed. Philadelphia, W.B. Saunders, 1994.
2. Davies D: Child Development: A Practitioner's Guide. New York, Guilford Press, 1999.
3. Downey G, Coyne JC: Children of depressed parents: An integrative review. Psychol Bull 108:50–76, 1990.
4. Fraiberg S: The Magic Years: Understanding and Handling the Problems of Early Childhood. New York, Scribner, 1959.
5. Fraiberg S, Adelson E, Shapiro V: Ghosts in the nursery: A psychoanalytic approach to the problems of impaired infant-mother relationships. J Am Acad Child Psychiatry 14:387–421, 1975.
6. Glascoe F: Early detection of developmental and behavioral problems. Pediatr Rev 21:272–279, 2000.
7. Green M, U.S. Maternal and Child Health Bureau, U.S. Medicaid Bureau, and National Center for Education in Maternal and Child Health: Bright Futures: Guidelines for Health Supervision of Infants, Children, and Adolescents. Arlington, VA, National Center for Education in Maternal and Child Health, 1994.
8. Kaplan-Sanoff M, Zuckerman B (eds): Healthy Steps Strategies for Change. Boston, Independent Production Fund, Toby Levine Communications, Inc., and Boston University School of Medicine Department of Pediatrics, 2000.
9. Wildey L, et al: Basic Concepts in Identifying the Health Need of Adolescents. Cincinnati, OH, Division of Adolescent Medicine, Center for Continuing Education in Adolescent Health, Children's Hospital Medical Center, 1994.

2. PHYSICAL ASSESSMENT OF THE INFANT AND CHILD

Barbara Hoyer Schaffner, PhD, RN, CPNP

1. Discuss the best general assessments of growth in children.

Height, weight, and head circumference (in children ≤ 2 years old) are considered the best indicators of health in children. Any one of these measurements should be viewed in relation to prior measurements of the child and to standardized measurements based on the physical growth charts compiled by the National Center for Health Statistics. Measurements of height and weight greater than the 97th percentile and less than the 3rd percentile for a child of that specific age and gender may indicate a growth disturbance and would require additional investigation by the clinician.

NEONATAL/INFANT ASSESSMENT

2. When is jaundice a dangerous sign in newborns?

Jaundice that develops within the first 24 hours of life or jaundice that persists beyond 2 weeks of life may be indicative of a hemolytic disease or biliary obstruction. Jaundice in an infant at any age that corresponds with other symptoms of illness and infection must be addressed aggressively.

3. Describe physiologic jaundice.

Physiologic, or normal, jaundice occurs in approximately 50% of infants. Physiologic jaundice appears on the second or third day of life, is at its worse during the fourth and fifth days of life, then subsides usually within 1 week, although some infants appear jaundiced for 30 days. Physiologic jaundice begins on the face and descends down the body. Jaundice that goes lower than the nipple level is worrisome, and further evaluation is needed.

4. List some risk factors of hyperbilirubinemia in the newborn.

Breast-feeding
Cephalhematoma
Too much water intake
Hemolytic disease
Infection

5. What is a cause of a jaundiced discoloration in older infants?

Older infants (usually ≥ 6 months old) may develop a jaundice (yellow-to-orange) color on the palms, soles, and nose but not sclera. In the absence of other signs of illness, this discoloration is caused by the ingestion of yellow vegetables (e.g., carrots, squash, and sweet potatoes) and is called **hypercarotenemia**.

6. Discuss common causes of swelling on the scalp of newborns.

The drawing of the scalp into the cervical os during labor and the trauma of birth cause **caput succedaneum**. It usually is found over the occiput and crosses suture lines. The swelling in the scalp usually subsides within the first 24 hours after birth.

Cephalhematomas are scalp swellings caused by subperiosteal hemorrhage within the first 24 hours of life. The swelling from cephalhematomas is characteristically firm with defined edges at initial presentation and enlarges for 2–3 days. It usually disappears within 2 weeks.

Although caput succedaneum and cephalhematomas look similar, the placement of the swelling across the newborn's suture lines makes the differentiation: Cephalhematomas do not cross the suture lines, whereas caput succedaneum can cross suture lines.

7. Describe the normal fontanels of infants.

Normal newborns have two fontanels in the anterior and posterior portion of the skull where the major sutures come together. Fontanels feel like soft concavities, or depressed ridges, and reflect intracranial pressure. The anterior fontanel is normally between 4 and 6 cm at its widest point at birth. The posterior fontanel is usually 1–2 cm at birth. Normally the anterior fontanel closes between 7 and 19 months (range, 4–26 months). The posterior fontanel closes between 2 and 3 months.

8. What is plagiocephaly?

The asymmetry that may develop in the appearance of an infant's scalp usually related to the infant's positioning during sleep time. Continuous positioning of an infant in the same position, usually on his or her back or side, during sleep time results in a **flattening** of the skull on the dependent side and a prominence on the opposite side. Normally, plagiocephaly disappears as the infant becomes more active or the positioning of the infant becomes more varied. In some severe cases, the infant is placed in a molding helmet to help reestablish the skull's normal shape, and rarely surgery is necessary.

9. Discuss interpretation of the Apgar score.

Apgar scores indicate an infant's immediate adaptation to the extrauterine environment. Scoring is done at 1 minute and 5 minutes after birth and rates the infant on a 3-point scale for heart rate, respiratory effort, muscle tone, reflex irritability, and color.

APGAR SCORE	INTERPRETATION
≤ 7 at 1 min	Nervous system depression
≤ 4 at 1 min	Severe newborn depression requiring immediate resuscitation
< 7 at 5 min	High risk of central nervous system or other system dysfunction

10. Explain Ballard scoring.

Ballard scoring is used to determine the newborn's maturity and gestational age in weeks. It assesses the newborn's neuromuscular and physical maturity.
- **Neuromuscular maturity** is rated based on posture, appearance of the wrist (square window), arm recoil, popliteal angle, the scarf sign, and heel-to-ear maneuver.
- **Physical maturity** is rated based on the extent of lanugo on the skin and appearance of the plantar surface, breasts, eyes and ears, and genitalia.
- The score is compared with **gestational age**:
  Small for gestational age
  Appropriate for gestational age
  Large for gestational age

Each category has its own differing mortality rate and identified incidence of postnatal health problems.

11. When is the best time to do a thorough newborn assessment?

2–3 hours after birth, a time when the examiner can expect good responsiveness from the newborn. Ideally, this initial extensive examination is completed 2–3 hours after a feeding.

12. Describe expected (normal) color changes in the newborn.

Acrocyanosis: Cyanosis of the hands and feet

Cutis marmorata: Transient mottling when the infant is exposed to cold

Erythema toxicum: A pink papular rash with vesicles on the thorax, back, and buttocks (appears approximately 24–48 hours after birth and disappears in several days)

Harlequin color changes: Color changes occurring when the infant lies on the side, with the dependent body parts pink and nondependent parts pale

Mongolian spots: Irregular areas of deep blue pigmentation usually in the sacral and gluteal areas; more predominant in African American and Native American infants and infants of Asian and Latin descent

Telangiectatic nevi (stork bites): Flat, deep pink localized areas usually seen on the back of the neck

13. Describe the Denver Developmental Screening Test II (DDST).

The DDST is the standard for measuring developmental milestones in infants and young children, from birth to 6 years of age. The DDST is not a measure of intelligence (IQ) but is designed to identify any developmental delays in the areas of speech, socialization, and fine and gross motor development. The DDST is easy to administer and is a relatively quick test. If the DDST suggests a delay or the examiner suspects a delay even with normal findings on the DDST, more sophisticated, sensitive tests should be administered.

VISION ASSESSMENT

14. When should visual acuity screening be started and with what measurement tools?

The visual acuity in **3-year-olds** is screened using the **Snellen E chart**. Charts with pictures instead of the E chart can be used if a child has difficulty identifying the direction of the E. Picture charts have not shown any special advantage in testing young children. It is sometimes necessary to have the child take home the eye chart for practice.

Visual acuity testing of children is conducted in schools. Nonetheless, visual acuity of children may change within a school year, and periodic eye screening during well-child examinations is recommended.

15. When should visual acuity approach 20/20?

Age 6 or 7 years.

16. Describe expected visual acuity before age 6 to 7 years.
- At birth, visual acuity is thought to be only light perception.
- At 3 years, visual acuity is ± 20/40.
- At 4–5 years, visual acuity is ± 20/30.

Any differences in acuity between the right and left eye are considered abnormal and should be referred to an ophthalmologist.

17. How should vision be assessed during infancy?

The presence or absence of visual reflexes, pupillary constriction to light, the red reflex, and blink reflex measure vision to some degree at birth. Holding the infant upright and rotating the infant slowly frequently helps to get the infant's eyes open.

Further assessments include **object fixation** at 2–4 months and **tracking** of an object at 5–6 months.

Ophthalmoscope examination usually is delayed until 2–6 months, when an infant is more cooperative, although the red reflex is present bilaterally at birth. Earlier examination of the red reflex is necessary if any of the ocular or neurologic examination is abnormal.

18. What are Brushfield's spots?

White spots scattered around the iris. They may be present in normal infants but in the presence of other physical findings may suggest Down's syndrome.

19. What is lazy eye?

A condition caused by **amblyopia**, reduced vision in an otherwise normal eye. It is the most prevalent eye disorder in early childhood, and treatment should begin at the time of diagnosis. With early intervention, amblyopia offers an excellent prognosis. Successful treatment is unlikely if treatment is begun after 6 years of age. The discovery of amblyopia at an early age emphasizes the need for visual screening of young children.

20. What assessment findings require immediate referral to an ophthalmologist?

AGE	SCREENING	REQUIRE FURTHER EVALUATION
≤ 3 mo	Red reflex	Abnormal
	Corneal light reflex	Asymmetric
	Inspection	Structural abnormality
6 mo–1 y	Red reflex	Abnormal
	Corneal light reflex	Asymmetric
	Fix and follow with each eye	Failure to fix and follow
3 y	Visual acuity	20/50 or worse
	Red reflex	Abnormal
	Corneal light reflex	Asymmetric
5 y	Visual acuity	20/30 or worse
	Red reflex	Abnormal
	Corneal light reflex	Asymmetric
	Inspection	Structural abnormality

EAR, NOSE, AND THROAT ASSESSMENT

21. Where should the external ear be located on the head?

Normal placement of the ears in relation to the face and scalp is with the upper portion of the auricle, the pinna, located as an extension of a line drawn across the inner and outer canthi of the eye. When the position of the ears is lower than expected or the ear is small in size, associated congenital anomalies should be suspected.

22. How and when should hearing be assessed in infants?

In the **first few days** of life, the parent's impression of the infant's hearing usually is accurate. A basic test of hearing in the young infant is the **acoustic blink reflex**. This reflex can be elicited by producing a sudden sharp noise about 12 inches from the infant's ear. A positive hearing response to a handclap or finger snap would be blinking of the eyes.

At about **2 weeks of age**, an infant should startle to loud noises; at 10 weeks, the infant may cease all movements for a moment when hearing a loud noise.

At approximately **3–4 months**, the infant should turn the head toward the sound stimuli.

At **6–10 months**, the infant should respond to his or her own name and the person's voice and localize sounds.

At **10–12 months**, the infant should recognize and localize sounds and should be imitating simple words and sounds.

23. How and when should hearing be assessed in children?

Simple auditory screening should be initiated with older children at all routine well-child visits. Simple auditory screening includes giving verbal commands and asking questions of the child. The **whisper test** can be used with hearing expected at approximately 12–24 inches.

24. In what children should brainstem auditory evoked response (BAER) testing be instituted?

In infants who are at high risk for hearing deficits, such as those with:
- A strong family history of hearing deficits
- Physical findings consistent with a hearing deficit
- Prenatal difficulties, such as low birth weight, anoxia, use of ototoxic medications, or exchange transfusions

- Congenital infections
- Hyperbilirubinemia (≥ 20 mg/dL)
- Meningitis

25. Describe the appearance of a normal tympanic membrane (TM).

A normal TM is pearly gray in color with a light reflex in the shape of a cone noticeable between 5:00 and 7:00 (picturing the TM as the face of a clock). The handle of the malleus should be visible descending through the center of the TM with the short process of the malleus superior to the handle. One difference of the TM in infancy is that the light reflex tends to be more diffuse and does not take on the characteristic cone shape for several months after birth.

26. Name two abnormal appearances of the TM and the conditions they may represent.

1. A red bulging TM usually is indicative of **acute otitis media**; an amber TM is associated with **serous otitis media**.

2. An unusually prominent short process of the malleus and a more prominent handle may suggest a **retracted eardrum**.

27. To visualize the TM in a child, how should the otoscopic examination be performed?

The speculum used on the otoscope should be of a size that provides comfort with a ¼- to ½-inch penetration into the external ear canal. Stabilization of the child's (or infant's) head is crucial for adequate visualization. When examining the right ear, turn the child's head to the left and hold firmly; do the opposite for examining the left ear.

- To visualize the TM in an infant, the examiner should pull the auricle gently downward.
- In the young child, the auricle is pulled upward, outward, and backward to view the TM.
- In older children and adolescents, the technique used with adults should be implemented, pulling the auricle upward and backward.

28. How should movement of the TM be checked during the otoscopic examination?

Pneumatic otoscopy is used. In the normal TM, the membrane and light reflex move inward with the introduction of air into the ear canal. Movement of the TM is diminished or absent with acute otitis media or serous otitis media.

29. How is nasal patency assessed in an infant?

Nasal patency must be assessed one nostril at a time. Many infants are obligatory nasal breathers, and obstructing both nares simultaneously leaves the infant unable to breathe. While occluding one naris, assess air movement through the other by feel of air movement or by use of a small piece of tissue placed under the naris and observing for the movement of the tissue. To confirm an obstructed nasal passage, attempt to pass a small-lumen catheter through each nostril into the posterior nasopharynx.

30. Which position is best to visualize the pharynx of an infant?

The supine position, using a source of light and a tongue blade. An adequate inspection of the pharynx can be completed in the infant and young child while crying.

31. Which position is best to visualize the pharynx of a child?

A child may be more comfortable and cooperative if held on the mother's lap. Elicit the help of the parent to hold the child's head still and hands down. If a tongue blade is needed, tickling the top of the palate frequently causes the child to open his or her mouth wider.

ORAL AND DENTAL ASSESSMENT

32. Discuss the significance of white spots found on the mucous membranes in the mouth.

White lacy spots on an erythematous base located along the oral mucous membranes may be oral *Candida* (**thrush**). An attempt should be made to differentiate thrush from milk curds left in the mouth from formula or milk. If the spots cannot be removed from the mucous membranes with a tongue blade or cotton applicator, the spots are thrush.

33. What does it mean when an infant begins drooling?

Saliva formation begins at about 3 months of age. Without lower teeth to serve as a dam to trap the saliva, the infant drools the secretions. At times of teething, the amount of oral secretions increases, again causing noticeable drooling.

34. When is tooth eruption expected?

There is a wide variation in age. African American children develop their teeth earlier than white infants.
- On average, a 10-month-old infant has two lower and two upper central incisors.
- A 2-year-old has 20 teeth.
- Shedding of primary teeth begins around 6 years of age.
- Eruption of permanent teeth occurs between the ages of 6 and 12 years.
- Development of permanent teeth continues through ages 17–22 years.

35. What is the most common cause of dental caries in infants?

Frequent consumption of carbohydrates. Nursing-bottle caries develops with prolonged bottle-feeding, especially with a nighttime bottle of milk or formula. When an infant falls asleep with a bottle, this allows carbohydrate-rich liquids to remain in the mouth and essentially bathe the teeth; this extensive contact causes decay of the primary teeth.

36. Name two sources of damage to the tooth enamel.

1. Irregular white specks on the enamel of children's teeth may result from excessive **fluoride intake**. Fluoride supplements should be given only to children whose drinking water supply is known to be without fluoride supplementation (e.g., well water that officially has been tested and found to be without fluoride or the child drinks exclusively fluoride-free bottled water).

2. **Tetracycline** given to children younger than 8 years may cause permanent graying of the permanent tooth enamel.

HEAD AND NECK ASSESSMENT

37. What is a common cause of snoring in young children?

Markedly enlarged adenoids or **tonsils**. Mouth breathing is frequently associated with snoring. In severe snoring conditions, the child may have irregular breathing patterns with the possibility of **sleep apnea**. A child who has severe snoring, restless sleep, and irregular breathing patterns should be referred to a specialist.

38. What is the relationship between sinus tenderness and sinusitis in children?

There is no definitive relationship. The complaint of headache, especially frontal headache, is common among children with infective sinusitis. When they approach adult size or around the teenage years, children with sinusitis may have associated tenderness over the sinus cavities on palpation.

39. Why are enlarged lymph nodes a more common finding in children than in adults?

The lymphatic system and lymphatic tissue grow in size much faster than the somatic growth of the child. Lymphatic tissue reaches adult size by age 4 years, exceeds adult size by 180% by age 10 years, then diminishes slowly to adult size by age 20 years. The excessive size of lymph tissue, especially in relation to the size of the child, makes enlarged lymph nodes more prevalent in children, especially children between the ages of 4 and 10 years, and more noticeable than in adults older than age 20 years.

40. When do enlarged lymph nodes warrant concern?

Lymph nodes smaller than 0.5 cm are not of concern. Nodes that have grown rapidly; are large (2–3 cm); or are painful, fixed, and immobile warrant further investigation.

41. Why do tonsils appear large in young children?

Similar to lymphatic tissue, tonsils in early and late childhood appear large in relation to the child's overall size. The size of the tonsils is exaggerated when the gag reflex is stimulated or the child says "ahh" and the tonsils move out of their fossae toward the midline of the throat. It frequently is said that tonsils reach their maximum size around age 4–5 years, and the child grows into the tonsils.

42. How are tonsils graded to describe their size?

GRADE	DESCRIPTION
1+	Visible
2+	Halfway between tonsillar pillars and uvula
3+	Nearly touching the uvula
4+	Touching each other

43. Discuss nuchal rigidity in infants and children.

Nuchal rigidity is characterized by a resistance to movement of the head and neck in any direction. It is an ominous sign and may indicate meningeal irritation from a central nervous system infection (**meningitis**), bleeding, or a tumor. Normally a child sitting upright should be able to touch the chest with the chin; with nuchal rigidity, such neck flexion is painful. Another way to detect nuchal rigidity is to have the examiner cradle the child's head in the hands while providing complete head support and attempt to move the head in all directions. A child with meningeal irritation actively resists the head movements.

RESPIRATORY ASSESSMENT

44. Describe normal respiratory patterns in newborns.

The normal breathing pattern is abdominal breathing in an irregular pattern at approximately 30–40 breaths/min. Periodic breathing, consisting of an irregular pattern with short periods of apnea, is common, especially in premature infants.

45. When are periods of apnea of significant concern in infants?

Periods of **apnea** that are greater than 20 seconds coupled with periods of bradycardia may indicate cardiopulmonary disease, central nervous system disease, or a high risk for **sudden infant death syndrome**.

46. Describe the difference between inspiratory wheezing and expiratory wheezing.

Inspiratory wheezing commonly is called **stridor** and may be indicative of upper airway disease, such as laryngotracheal bronchitis (**croup**).

Expiratory wheezing usually indicates narrowing of the lower airway passages and is more consistent with reactive airway disease (**asthma**).

47. How does the appearance of the infant and young child's chest differ from that of an adult?

The infant's chest has a **barreled** appearance, similar to the **adult barrel chest** seen with chronic obstructive pulmonary disease. In the barrel chest appearance of the infant, the transverse to anteroposterior diameter, thoracic index, is 1. The appearance of the child's chest becomes more adultlike at approximately 6 years of age, with a thoracic index of 1.35.

48. List the differences in the child's respiratory system compared with the respiratory system in adults.
- Thin chest wall allows breath sounds to sound louder and harsher.
- Soft pliable chest wall allows for more visible use of accessory muscles and retractions.
- Decreased number of alveoli makes children more susceptible to respiratory distress with pulmonary disease.
- Obligatory nose breathing allows for compromised respiration with nasal congestion and upper respiratory illnesses.
- Large-sized tongue in relation to oropharynx increases chances of airway obstruction.
- Weaker cough diminishes the normal cleaning mechanism of the body to protect the respiratory system.
- Narrow airways allow increased respiratory distress with swelling and inflammation of any of the upper and lower respiratory structures.

THORAX ASSESSMENT

49. Why do the breasts of male and female newborns appear enlarged?
The influence of maternal estrogen causes an enlargement of the breast tissue. The breasts may be enlarged and even engorged with a white liquid at birth, sometimes referred to as **witch's milk**. Enlargement of the breasts usually disappears in about 2 weeks and rarely lasts beyond 3 months.

50. Where is the point of maximal impulse (PMI) found in infants and children?
The PMI is visible in infants and children at the fourth **intercostal space (ICS)** left of the midclavicular line. By age 7 years, the PMI has descended to the fifth ICS. The PMI remains left of the midclavicular line until approximately age 4 years, becomes midclavicular around age 4–6 years, and is found right of the midclavicular line by age 7 years.

CARDIOPULMONARY ASSESSMENT

51. List signs of severe heart disease in children.
- Poor weight gain
- Delayed development
- Tachypnea
- Tachycardia
- Heaving or thrusting precordium
- Cyanosis
- Clubbing of the nails

52. Is an innocent, or benign, heart murmur a common diagnosis?
Yes; 50% of children are diagnosed with an innocent murmur.

53. List the characteristics of an innocent murmur.
- Systolic
- Short duration
- Less than 3/6 intensity
- Low-pitched
- Vibratory
- Loudest at the fourth ICS, medial to the apex
- Poorly transmitted
- Intensity changes with positional changes
- Heard better in high–cardiac output states, such as fever and exercise

54. Do blood pressure readings taken in the arms and legs of children usually differ?

Yes, with the blood pressure measured in the thigh being approximately 10 mmHg higher than the blood pressure measured in the upper arm. As the child grows, this difference disappears.

55. When is a difference in blood pressure readings taken in the arms and legs of children of clinical concern?

If the **thigh blood pressure** is found to be **lower** than the blood pressure taken in the upper arm, the existence of a **coarctation of the aorta** must be considered and investigated.

56. How are blood pressure readings in children recorded?

Readings are recorded with the systolic reading being the **Korotkoff 1 sound**, when the tapping noise begins. The diastolic reading is recorded in accordance with the **Korotkoff 5 sound**, the disappearance of sound.

57. What size blood pressure cuff should be used in children?

The width of the blood pressure cuff should measure 90% of the circumference of the limb being measured. Too narrow a cuff produces a falsely elevated blood pressure, whereas a too-wide cuff produces a falsely low blood pressure. The bladder of the blood pressure cuff should be long enough to encircle 80–100% of the limb being measured.

58. List congenital heart diseases that cause cyanosis and those that do not.

ACYANOTIC HEART DISEASE	CYANOTIC HEART DISEASE
Patent ductus arteriosus	Tetralogy of Fallot
Atrial septal defect	Tricuspid atresia
Ventricular septal defect	Transposition of the great vessels
Pulmonic stenosis	Two- and three- chambered hearts
Aortic stenosis	
Coarctation of the aorta	

Pearl: Congenital heart diseases that begin with the letter *T* tend to be cyanotic defects.

ABDOMINAL ASSESSMENT

59. Describe the normal appearance of vessels in the umbilicus of a newborn.

Three vessels normally appear, two thick-walled arteries and one thin-walled vein. The vein normally is visible at the 12:00 position and tends to be wider in diameter than the two arteries.

60. What is the significance of the occurrence of a single umbilical artery?

If a single artery is present, the chance of the infant having a **congenital anomaly** is high.

61. Describe the appearance of a healthy healing umbilicus.

The umbilicus consists of two portions, the umbilicus cutis and umbilicus amnioticus. The umbilicus cutis is cutaneous and covered with skin. The skin of the umbilicus cutis retracts into the abdominal wall and becomes the navel. The umbilicus amnioticus is the amniotic portion and is covered by a gelatin-type substance. The umbilicus amnioticus normally dries up in approximately 1 week and falls off in about 2 weeks. Daily application of rubbing alcohol to the base of the umbilicus promotes drying and removal of the umbilicus amnioticus.

62. In what order is the abdominal assessment performed?

1. Inspection
2. Auscultation
3. Percussion
4. Light palpation
5. Deep palpation

63. How does percussion of the abdomen differ in infants from adults?

Infants tend to swallow more air during feeding and crying, and there tends to be distention of the abdomen and intestinal lumen, which sounds tympanic on percussion.

64. What is the normal liver span percussed in differing aged children?

AGE (YR)	MEAN LIVER SPAN (CM)	
	MALES	FEMALES
0.5 (6 mo)	2.4	2.8
1	2.8	3.1
2	3.5	3.6
3	4.0	4.0
4	4.4	4.3
5	4.8	4.5
6	5.1	4.8
8	5.6	5.1
10	6.1	5.4
12	6.5	5.6
14	6.8	5.8
16	7.1	6.0
18	7.4	6.1
20	7.7	6.3

From Hoekelman RA: The physical examination of infants and children. In Bickley LS, Hoekelman RA (eds): Bates Guide to Physical Examination and History Taking, 7th ed. Philadelphia, J.B. Lippincott, 1999.

65. List assessment findings that would be consistent with a surgical abdomen.

Marked abdominal distention
Abdominal tenderness
Increased pitch and frequency of bowel sounds
Rebound tenderness
Guarding
Knee-chest positioning
Absence of defecation

GENITOURINARY ASSESSMENT

66. Where is the urethral orifice located in normal male infants and in male infants with hypospadias?

• In normal infants, at the end of the penile shaft
• In infants with **hypospadias**, on the ventral surface of the glans or shaft of the penis

67. Is scrotal edema normal in newborn boys?

Yes. Scrotal edema is present in newborn males for several days after birth because of the influence of maternal estrogen.

68. When is scrotal edema cause for clinical concern?

If scrotal edema lasts more than a couple of days, it may be due to a **hydrocele**. Transillumination of the scrotum reveals the excess fluid. Most hydroceles reabsorb spontaneously by 18 months of age.

69. Describe the assessment of the scrotal sac.

The scrotum in male infants appears large compared with the rest of the genitalia. Testicles can be palpated in the scrotal sac. To assess scrotal content in older boys, have the boys in a sitting position with their legs crossed.

70. What is cryptorchidism?

Undescended testicles, which affects 3% of infants. By 1 year of age, most undescended testicles have descended spontaneously.

71. Is genital edema normal in newborn girls?

Yes. Prominence of the mons pubis, labia majora, and labia minora is common at birth because of the influence of maternal estrogen. The hymen tends to be thick and protruding. Edema usually disappears by approximately 2 weeks after birth.

72. Describe the changes of puberty in boys.

Changes do not occur at exactly the same time in each boy. The Tanner chart shows pubertal development. The development of genital and pubic hair is related to age and evidence of a height spurt. External genital changes usually come before pubic hair. Ejaculation generally occurs at stage 3 with semen appearing about stage 3 to 4.

Tanner Stages for Males

TANNER STAGE	PUBIC HAIR DEVELOPMENT	PENIS SCROTUM DEVELOPMENT
1	No hair growth	No change in size or shape
2	Slightly pigmented long straight hair, usually at base of penis	Enlargement of scrotum and testes
3	Dark pigmented curly pubic hair around base of penis	Enlargement of penis in length, enlargement of testes, descent of scrotum
4	Pubic hair definitely adult in type but not extent	Continued enlargement of penis, increased pigmentation of scrotum
5	Hair spread to medial surface of thighs	Scrotum ample, penis reaching to bottom of scrotum

73. Describe the changes of puberty in girls.

Changes do not occur at exactly the same time in each girl. The Tanner chart shows pubertal development. The stage and rate of breast development and pubic hair development are related to chronologic age, age of menarche, and height spurt. Breasts begin to develop before pubic hair in most girls. Menarche usually begins around breast stage 3 to 4, and sexual maturity occurs at stage 4. The peak height spurt in girls usually occurs before menarche.

Tanner Stages for Females

TANNER STAGE	PUBIC HAIR DEVELOPMENT	BREAST DEVELOPMENT
1	No growth	Only nipple is raised
2	Initial sparse straight hair,	Budding stage, areola increased in diameter
3	Sparse, dark curly pubic hair on labia	Breast and areola enlarged, no contour separation
4	Hair coarse and curly, less than adult	Increasing fat deposits. Areola forms above breast
5	Lateral spreading into adult triangular pattern	Adult appearance, nipple projects
6	Extension laterally, upward	

74. What about delayed onset of adolescence and puberty?

Delayed onset is often a normal variable in boys and girls. When the pubertal changes begin, the sequence of development is the same for all adolescents but may occur over a shorter period of time.

75. What characteristics are consistent with precocious puberty?

- In girls, the existence of pubic hair or breast enlargement or both before age 8 years
- In boys, sexual development, with beginning pubic hair and enlargement of the scrotum and testes, before age 9 years

76. Name characteristics that indicate ambiguous genitalia in a newborn.

Enlarged clitoris
Fusion of the labia majora

77. How should the sex of the child with ambiguous genitalia be determined?

By hormonal and genetic analysis.

78. Is vaginal discharge normal during adolescence?

Yes. Physiologic **leukorrhea**, which is a whitish vaginal discharge, is common in adolescent girls. Drainage that becomes purulent may indicate a foreign body in the vagina.

79. Describe a routine genitalia examination in a girl.

For general purposes, an external genitalia examination is adequate for prepubertal girls. A recommended position is lying supine in the frog-legged position.

80. What circumstances indicate a need for an internal genitalia examination?

- Suspicions of sexual abuse
- Vaginal bleeding in a prepubertal girl

81. List red flags that may indicate sexual abuse.

- Evidence of overall abuse or neglect
- Evidence of trauma in genital, anal, and perianal areas
- Unusual changes in skin color or pigmentation in genital or anal area
- Presence of sexually transmitted disease
- Anorectal problems
- Genitourinary problems
- Behavioral problems, such as sexually provocative mannerisms, excessive sexual knowledge, and excessive masturbation
- Significant behavioral changes in school, eating patterns, or sleeping patterns

82. What are indications for a rectal examination in pediatric patients?

Suspicion of intra-abdominal, pelvic, or perirectal disease.

MUSCULOSKELETAL ASSESSMENT

83. What observation may help differentiate true deformities of the musculoskeletal system from positional differences in infants?

Intrauterine position of the newborn may account for the abnormal appearance of a limb. Positional differences without true deformity allow for complete manipulation of the joint through all planes of movement. A true deformity does not return to a neutral position with manipulation.

84. Describe the position of the foot when talipes equinovarus (clubfoot) is present.

The forefoot is adducted and inverted with plantar flexion of the entire foot. The clubfoot cannot be manipulated to a normal and neutral position.

85. Discuss bowleg and knock knee.

Bowleg (genu varum) is a common finding of toddlers until the age of 18 months. Bowleg is a space between the knees of 1 inch. Many children with genu varum as infants progress to **knock knee (genu valgum)** from age 2 years until age 4 years. Genu valgum is a 1-inch space between the medial malleoli. Most children with genu varum and genu valgum straighten without intervention. Assessment for genu varum and genu valgum should be made with the child standing with the knees at the level of the examiner's vision.

86. How and when should infants' hips be examined for hip dislocation?

The hips of all infants should be assessed for dislocation. To obtain the **Ortolani sign**, flex the legs to right angles at the hips and knees and place index fingers over the greater trochanter of each femur and thumbs over the lesser trochanters. Abduct both hips simultaneously until the lateral aspect of each knee touches the examination table. With hip dislocation, a **click** can be heard and a **clunk** felt as the femoral head enters the acetabulum during the 90° abduction. Beyond the newborn period, at about 2 months, the increase in strength of the hip muscles makes the Ortolani sign less obtainable. After 2 months of age, the best sign of a dislocated hip is decreased abduction of the flexed leg, unequal leg length, and unequal gluteal folds of the thigh and buttocks.

87. How is hip disease identified in an older child?

In the Trendelenburg test, with the child standing on one foot, the pelvis should remain level; with hip disease, the pelvis tilts. Leg shortening, one leg shorter than the other, is another sign of hip disease.

88. Describe screening for scoliosis.

The child should bend forward touching the toes. The clinician should examine the spine from behind, assessing for symmetry of the scapulae, rib cage, and hip. The clinician may elicit a complaint of uneven fitting of clothes from the child or family.

NEUROLOGIC ASSESSMENT

89. How can mental status be evaluated from infancy through adolescence?

- In **infancy**, mentation is assessed by observing the ease of transition of the infant from alertness to drowsiness and the ease of consolability.
- In **older infants**, mentation is assessed by observing the recognition of significant others.
- In **toddlers**, mentation is assessed by observing the recognition of significant objects.
- In **preschoolers**, mentation is assessed through the verbalization and understanding of language.
- In **children ages 4-6 years old**, beginning problem-solving abilities can be assessed using such questions as "what would you do if you were outside playing and got hungry?"; "what would you do if you got cold?".
- In **school-age children**, math and reading skills can be assessed and memory tasks, such as recall of last meal, repeating of a seven-digit number.
- In **adolescents**, abstract reasoning can be assessed through the interpretation of parables.

90. Describe assessment of gross and fine motor development.

Assessment of motor development can be accomplished through range of motion of each joint and assessment of muscle tone. The **DDST** can be used to evaluate the gross and fine motor skills of a child compared with norms for the child's age. Abnormal positioning of the body, asymmetry, and extension of the extremities and head must be considered signs of possible intracranial disease.

91. How are sensory assessments of infants and children conducted
- **Infants** should withdraw from noxious stimulation, such as flicking of the hands or feet.
- **Older children** can be tested for thresholds of pain, touch, and temperature.

92. Describe cranial nerve assessment in infants and young children.

CRANIAL NERVE	NEWBORN/INFANT	YOUNG CHILDREN
II Optic	Optical blink reflex	Snellen E or picture chart
III Oculomotor	Gazes intently at an object	Tracking an object
IV Trochlear VI Abducens	Tracks an object with both eyes	Move the object through the cardinal fields of gaze
V Trigeminal	Rooting reflex Sucking reflex	Chewing Touch forehead with cotton and have child bat away
VII Facial	Observe expression when crying	Observe face when smiling, crying, frowning
VIII Acoustic	Acoustic blink reflex Moves eyes in direction of sound	Turns to sounds Repeats whispered word Audiometric testing
IX Glossopharyngeal	Swallowing reflex Gag reflex	Elicit gag reflex
X Vagus	Swallowing reflex	Swallowing Quality of speech sounds
XI Spinal accessory	Coordinated sucking and swallowing	Stick out tongue Shrug shoulders/raise arms
XII Hypoglossal	Pinch nose, infant opens mouth and mouths tongue upward	Tongue protrusion, symmetry, and strength

93. Describe the appearance, characteristics, and disappearance of infant reflexes.

REFLEX	APPEARANCE	DISAPPEARANCE
Babinski (plantar)	Birth	16–24 mo
Palmar grasp	Birth	3–4 mo
Rooting	Birth	3–4 mo
Moro	Birth	6 mo
Placing	Approximately 4 days	Varies
Stepping	Birth–8 wk	Before walking
Fencing	By 2–3 mo	Diminishes at 3–4 mo; disappears at 6 mo

CONTROVERSY

94. Is there a difference in the expected growth of breast-fed infants versus formula-fed infants?

It generally is found that breast-fed infants tend to fall in the lower percentiles on the National Center for Health Statistics growth charts for weight and height. Some child health experts have suggested that these lower growth percentiles have contributed to a lower rate of breast-feeding in the United States. Because the breast-fed infant is labeled as small in relation to other infants, the fear that the breast-fed infant is not getting enough milk intensifies. The concern of inadequate nutrition for the breast-fed infant is compounded by societal pressure to ensure adequate food for the infant and the image of the pudgy infant as a healthy infant. Some experts have suggested that separate growth charts be developed for breast-fed infants. Showing through breast-fed–specific growth charts that the infant is growing normally might provide an added incentive to mothers and families to continue breast-feeding infants for as long as possible.

BIBLIOGRAPHY

1. Augustine MC: Hyperbilirubinemia in the healthy term newborn. Nurse Pract 24:24–26, 29–32, 1999.
2. Bacal DA, Rousta ST, Hertle RW: Why early vision screening matters. Contemp Pediatr 16:155, 1999.
3. Bickley LS, Hoekelman RA: Bates Guide to Physical Examination and History Taking, 7th ed. Philadelphia, Lippincott Williams & Wilkins, 1999.
4. Henry JJ: Routine growth monitoring and assessment of growth disorders. J Pediatr Health Care 6:291, 1996.
5. Hobbie C, Baker S, Bayerl C: Parental understanding of basic infant nutrition: Misinformed feeding choices. J Pediatr Health Care 14:26–31, 2000.
6. Kaleida PH: The COMPLETES exam for otitis. Contemp Pediatr 14:93, 1997.
7. Leder MR, Knight JR, Emans SJ: Sexual abuse: When to suspect it, how to assess for it. Contemp Pediatr 18:59, 2001.
8. Seidel HM, Ball JW, Dains JE, Benedict TW: Mosby's Guide to Physical Examination, 4th ed. St. Louis, Mosby, 1999.
9. Smith KM: The innocent heart murmur in children. J Pediatr Health Care 11:207–214, 1997.
10. Verst A: Get in the game: Principles of the preparticipation physical. Adv Nurse Pract 8:66–68, 2000.
11. Wong DL: Nursing Care of Infants and Children, 6th ed. St. Louis, Mosby, 1999.

3. PARENTING AND ISSUES RELATED TO CHILD ABUSE

Bruce K. Wilson, PhD

1. Should nurses focus on the family in addition to the problems of the child?

Yes. The child is like a young plant. The nurse can see only the part sticking above the ground. The child draws most of his or her strength and nourishment from the root structure (the family), which is hidden beneath the surface. The more we can help provide a healthy environment for the root structure, the stronger and healthier the child will grow. Numerous research studies show that the better the family functions as a unit and the better the family members communicate with each other, the healthier the children are physiologically, psychologically, and socially.

2. Don't parents know how to care for their child?

When a child is born, there is no attached instruction manual, and the parents are not infused suddenly with all necessary knowledge. Parents often attend childbirth classes, but they do not take any classes for child rearing. The pediatric nurse should play a major role in assessing the family environment and providing necessary guidance.

3. What kind of guidance should the nurse provide to parents?

A major part of the guidance is helping the parents protect the child from injury. **Injury** is the major cause of death in children. Parents should be directed to sources for home safety materials. The **American Heart Association** is an inexpensive source of written information. The nurse should try to spend at least as much time discussing what the parents are doing right as pointing out where improvements need to be implemented. Questions such as, "How have you changed your home to make it safer for your child?" help start the discussion in a positive tone.

4. Describe a healthy family environment.

A healthy family is flexible, allows each member to grow and change, and sees each individual member as multifaceted. **Flexibility** permits the family to work through various triumphs and adversities. None of the individual family members is constrained to a single role or function. Children are given additional appropriate responsibilities and privileges as they mature. The family is able to maintain flexibility in adapting to changes, while providing a **consistency** of expectations, affection, support, and mutual respect toward each other. No family functions perfectly all the time.

5. How should nurses approach nontraditional families?

Nursing activity should be directed at making a physically and psychologically safe environment for the child, rather than molding the environment to the nurse's preconceptions.

Most families are not the traditional middle-class construct of a married mother and father and 2.5 children. In this chapter, the term *parents* means the adults providing long-term physical, emotional, and spiritual support to the child. Parents may have different child-rearing practices.

6. Give examples of nontraditional families.

A single parent
A couple of the same gender
More than two adults in an extended family

7. How can the nurse help parents deal with a child's problem behaviors?

The nurse always should start with assessing the child and the family environment. Even children within the same family respond differently. Some children stop immediately when told to stop, whereas others run faster to accomplish what they want before a parent stops them. If a child has a strong-willed temperament, parents need to work harder to keep the child safe.

8. List items to consider when assessing a child's problem behavior.

1. The child's development
2. The child's temperament
3. Whether the behavior is harmful to the child or others

9. Discuss how parents can handle temper tantrums.

Temper tantrums are most common when a child is unable to get what he or she wants and tend to increase when the child is tired. Most temper tantrums are handled best by ignoring them. Giving in to a temper tantrum is telling the child that temper tantrums are a way of getting what the child wants. If the environment is contributing to the situation, the child should be removed to a calmer place. Parents may need to be reassured that children will not hurt themselves by holding their breath. Some children bang their head during tantrums. This behavior is normally self-limited, and the banging does not result in bruising.

10. Describe strategies parents can use if the child's behaviors harm the child or others.

Through the preschool years, children do not see others as individuals and may hit, bite, or scratch to get what they want. They need to be given a clear message that the behavior is not permitted, and they should be watched and restrained from the behavior in the future. Restraint works much better than physically punishing the child. If children are physically punished, they may learn that causing physical pain is a method to get wants met. If children are restrained, they do not get what they want, and they learn that biting, hitting, and scratching do not get them what they want.

11. What about the child who is a picky eater?

Unless there is some underlying disorder, children will not starve themselves. Struggles over eating cause stress in both the parent and the child and lead to more conflicts. Frequently, children do not like the same foods as adults. Generally, it is best to let the child have some options of relatively healthy foods. A low-sugar cereal and low-fat milk may be an easy meal for the picky eater. If the parents are concerned about the child's nutrition, a vitamin supplement can be given.

12. How should a parent manage a child with obesity?

The best solution is increasing the amount of exercise the child gets. Obese children tend not to be physically active, which increases the obesity, which leads to further decreases in activity.

13. Discuss sleep problems.

One of the differences between childhood and adulthood is that adults fight to take naps and children fight not to take naps. With preschool children, telling them they do not have to go to sleep at naptime but just lie quietly for half an hour relieves the pressure of having to sleep. Bedtime rituals (e.g., bath, brush teeth, say prayers, have a story read) help the child relax at the end of the day. When a child is hospitalized, it is important to follow the same pattern the child follows at home.

14. What should parents do if a child regresses to earlier behaviors?

When children feel stress, they frequently regress to earlier behaviors. A toilet-trained child suddenly may start wetting his or her pants, or a child may start needing a security item that previously was discarded. If this behavior is **tolerated** through the stressful period, the child soon will stop the regressive behavior. Focusing on the behavior adds to the child's stress and may prolong the regression.

15. When should families be encouraged to seek counseling for problem behaviors?

Parents should seek external assistance when their actions are not accomplishing the desired response in their child. The child may be experiencing physical or psychological imbalances that can be corrected easily, or the parents may need to try a different approach. Parents also should seek external help when there is a sudden unexplained change in the child's behavior.

16. What is the first step in evaluating a child with behavioral problems?

A complete battery of physiologic tests. Many physiologic imbalances are treated easily.

17. Describe dysfunctional families.

Members of dysfunctional families tend to view one another in terms of limiting roles, instead of complex human beings. Family members are restricted to these roles, which limit the individual's growth and the growth of the family as a unit. The family rigidity requires members to stay in these roles in an erroneous belief that the family would not exist without the roles. These families tend to become increasingly dysfunctional as they try to solve their problems by increasing the dysfunctional behavior. Dysfunctional families frequently are isolated from the community and have few social ties outside the immediate family. The lack of a relationship with the community reinforces the dysfunction, which in turn isolates the family further. The family members tend to form tight bonds with one another and work to protect the family secrets from the outside world. It is common in cases in which child abuse is proved for some family members to continue to deny that the abuse occurred. The abused child may take the blame for the abuse and express guilt for causing the parent to get "in trouble."

18. What is one source of dysfunctional families?

A mismatch between the characteristics of the child and the characteristics of the parents. A hyperactive child or seriously ill child may restrict the parents' ability to interact with the greater community. An infant who is not cuddly or is irritable may frustrate the parents' desire or need for a loving child.

19. What happens to children from dysfunctional families as they become adults?

Individuals growing up in abusive environments tend to form dysfunctional families as adults. Not all child abusers grew up in abusive homes, and not all individuals who grew up in abusive homes become child abusers. Because children who have grown up in dysfunctional families have not learned how healthy parents function, however, they have a much more difficult time functioning as parents.

20. Describe some typical dysfunctional child roles.

The hero. The task of the hero child is to provide hope for the entire family. The child is expected to accomplish some great task that somehow saves the family. Typically, these tasks are athletic or academic. The child has the burden of being required to save the entire family. The family focus is on supporting and encouraging only this member.

The scoundrel. The scoundrel is just the opposite of the hero. This child's task is always to be viewed as bad. By being perceived as the problem, this child provides the focus for the family's negative feelings.

The missing or lost child. This child adapts to the dysfunctional family by disappearing. Frequently, the child hides from the family for extended periods under the bed or in a closet. The family ignores the child's accomplishments, good or bad.

The comedian. The task of this child is to divert attention from the real problems the family is facing. The use of humor diffuses tension, but also distracts the family from solving their problems.

21. Define a healthy view of a child.

A sometimes good, sometimes bad, sometimes funny, sometimes needing privacy, emerging, loved human being.

22. Describe some typical dysfunctional adult roles.

The martyr. The martyr sacrifices his or her existence in an attempt to preserve the family. The martyr resents having to make sacrifices and refuses to share the responsibility with the other family members. Because the martyr does not share responsibility, other family members do not learn to be responsible.

The amusement park parent. The parent attempts to purchase the child's love and happiness. The parent fails to understand that children are most secure when there is a mixture of play, work, and rest. This behavior is seen frequently in cases of divorce with the noncustodial parent, but also may be seen in parents with an ill child.

The disciplinarian. The parent sees his or her task as forcing the other family members to follow a fixed set of rules.

The inconsistent parent. The parent reacts differently at various times to the same behavior. Family members are unable to clarify the expected consequences of behavior because the parental response keeps changing. Identical behavior at one time may be rewarded and at another time be punished.

23. How should a nurse work with difficult parents?

The primary skill in working with parents is to listen to their concerns. A conversation can be initiated by looking at the parent and stating, "You've had a difficult day haven't you?" Any day a parent has to take a child to a health care setting is a difficult day. Healthy parents discuss their concerns about their child. If the parent talks about all the other things in his or her life that are going wrong, the nurse should become suspicious of a potential child abuse situation.

24. List the types of abuse.

Emotional abuse
Neglect
Physical abuse
Sexual abuse

25. What are some general facts about child abuse?
- Within the family, only one child may be abused or several or all of the children.
- The child may be subjected to all the different types of abuse.
- A common misconception is that the abusive parent does not want the child. In fact, the parent wants the child but for the wrong reasons.

26. State a statistic that reflects the incidence of child abuse.

In the United States in 1998, 903,000 children were identified as victims of child abuse. This is a rate of 12.9 victims for each 1000 children.

27. Describe emotional abuse.

Emotional abuse generally is not recognized under the legal definition of child abuse. Many adults who were victims of severe child abuse describe the emotional abuse as more painful than the physical abuse. Emotional abuse inflicts psychological scars on the child victim. Abusive behaviors include belittling the child, telling the child that he or she is worthless, and telling the child that he or she has caused the adult's problems. Emotional abuse steals childhood from the child. The child is expected to act as an adult, with the physical, mental, and emotional strength of an adult. Childhood emotional abuse leaves the individual with a sense of shame and a lack of self-worth. Emotionally abused children may be given too many restrictions or too few restrictions. A child needs boundaries appropriate for the stage of development.

28. Define child neglect.

This is the most common type of child abuse. In 1998, according to the National Child Abuse and Neglect Data System, about 55% of the total victims were subjected to physical or medical neglect. **Physical neglect** is failing to provide the child's basic physiologic needs, such as food, water, shelter, or hygienic needs. Failure to provide necessary medical care is classified as **medical neglect**. Neglect also includes leaving the child in an unsafe environment.

29. Give an example of neglect involving an unsafe environment.

Leaving a 6-year-old child in charge of his or her younger siblings for an extended period.

30. What is failure to thrive?

Neglected infants fail to develop normally in the home environment. When their physical condition is stabilized in the hospital, they start gaining weight. If these infants are sent home, they stop progressing again. Home visits are a necessary part of the follow-up care to cases without an identified cause.

31. Describe the characteristics of neglecting parents.

1. Female parents commit more than 50% of the cases of physical neglect, and both parents commit about 17%.

2. Homeless families are not able to meet their children's needs.

3. Some families are unable to provide food for their children.

4. Some parents may believe that they cannot afford proper medical care, resulting in medical neglect. Even with insurance, a visit to the physician may cause major disruption to the family's budget.

32. Define physical abuse.

Causing severe physical damage to a child.

33. How can the nurse assist parents in learning methods other than physical punishment for controlling their child?

- Helping the parent identify the child's ability for **self-control**. If a child lacks the maturity for self-control, the child will be able to master the task only when he or she gains the maturity. Hitting the child will not make the child mature faster.
- Identifying other methods of helping the child to control his or her own behavior. If the child is incapable of self-control and that limitation poses a hazard to the child or another, **external controls** are appropriate. For example, if there is a firearm in the house, it should be kept in a manner that a child could not possibly gain access to the firearm.

34. List methods parents can use to control a child's behavior.

The best learning experience for a child occurs when the behavior is linked to a **consequence.** If a child is hitting another with a truck, the child is not permitted to play with the truck for a period of time. All consequences should be for a limited period. If a child is told that the penalty for taking a cookie without permission is never to get another cookie, the child is told that the only way to get a cookie is to take it without permission.

The child needs to be told which **alternative behaviors** are appropriate. A child who is told to lie down for 30 minutes should be give the option of sleeping or just resting quietly. If the child is told only "to take a nap," the child may become so concerned about falling asleep that he or she becomes unable to sleep.

Parents should spend more time **reinforcing the child's appropriate behavior** than trying to stop inappropriate behavior.

Child control should not be linked to how the child's behavior makes the parent feel. The child's task is not to control the parent's feelings.

In all methods of child control, the child should be loved, respected, and valued as a person. Children need to be secure in the knowledge that their parent values them regardless of their behavior.

35. When should the nurse be alert to the possibility of physical abuse?
Physical abuse should be considered in all cases of childhood trauma. The nurse always must compare the physical findings with the history provided by the caregiver and whenever possible a history from the child. In cases of child abuse, the physical assessment findings frequently do not match the history.

36. List signs of physical abuse.
Spiral fractures
Multiple fractures in various stages of healing
Bruises of various ages
A pattern of circular marks from cigarette burns
Linear scarring on the buttocks and legs
Scalding that does not fit the typical pattern

37. Explain what is meant by a typical pattern of injury.
Accidental injuries generally do not result in regular-shaped burns or bruising. A child who accidentally put his or her hands in hot water would automatically jerk them away, resulting in an irregular burn pattern, not a uniform burn to both hands stopping at the wrist. A stun gun injury results in a pair of circular lesions about 2 inches apart.

38. What is shaken baby syndrome?
A type of physical abuse that occurs when a caretaker shakes an infant. An infant has weak neck vertebrae and a weak support structure for the brain. Shaking an infant causes the brain to move within the skull, tearing it away from the fragile support structures. An examination of the retina may indicate a possible shaken infant. Radiologic studies of the head and spinal taps show the damage.

39. What are other indications of physical abuse?
• The child who does not respond in an age-appropriate manner to painful procedures may be a victim of abuse. For example, a 4-year-old who holds his arm out still and does not cry when blood is being drawn should raise suspicion.
• Abused children are sometimes protective of their parents. The child may comfort the parent in situations in which a parent normally would be comforting the child.
• The child may be dressed in a way that does not match the situation described by the child and the parents.

40. What is Munchausen syndrome by proxy?
Caregivers with this syndrome purposely cause a child to become ill or more severely ill. In some cases, the parent may withhold required medications. For example, in a child with a seizure disorder, the parent may withhold the anticonvulsive medications. In other cases, the caregiver may give inappropriate medications or deliberately introduce infectious agents into the child.

41. List cultural healing practices that may appear as physical abuse.
• C'ao gio—In this Vietnamese practice, fluid is applied to the chest or back and rubbed with a coin or shell, leaving a distinctive pattern.
• Cupping or spoon rubbing—This practice leaves circular marks on the trunk of the child's body.
• Maqua—In some parts of Africa and the Middle East, hot metal is applied to the site of injury or disease, leaving deep burns.

• **Moxibustion**—In some Asian cultures, herbs are burned at specific areas on the skin, leaving behind acute burns.

42. Name two instances of cultural or religious practices that are considered child abuse.

1. "Female circumcision" (female genital mutilation) is illegal in the United States and Canada.

2. In 2001, a Christian minister and some members of a congregation in Atlanta, Georgia, were charged with child abuse for severely beating children in the congregation.

43. List physiologic conditions that may present with symptoms similar to child abuse.

A variety of **bone diseases** may cause fractures. A spiral fracture is usually the result of a twisting force not an orthopedic disorder.

Hematologic disorders may cause bruising that initially appears as possible battering. Other skin disorders, such as mongolian spots, which is a bluish pigmentation on the lower back or upper buttocks, may be mistaken for a bruise.

Contact dermatitis may cause unusual skin disorders. The pattern of the skin disturbance provides clues to the causative agent.

Sudden infant death syndrome occurs in infants younger than 1 year old. These children frequently appear to be battered, and resuscitation efforts may add to the confusion. An autopsy should be conducted to determine the cause of death, and there may be a further investigation at the location where the infant died.

44. What is sexual abuse?

Using a child to provide sexual pleasure to an adult.

45. Describe misconceptions about child sexual abuse.

MISCONCEPTION	FACT
Only intercourse counts as sexual abuse.	Sexual abuse includes a wide variety of sexual behaviors in addition to intercourse.
Sexual abuse is committed only by the child's father	Fathers acting alone commit only 22% of the cases of child abuse. Mothers, other relatives, and other adults also commit sexual abuse.
Only girls are sexually abused.	Both boys and girls are sexually abused. Sexual abuse of boys may be substantially underreported because of social pressures. Because individuals other than family members often abuse boys, boys may be afraid to report the abuse.
The child caused the abuse.	Children who are abused frequently falsely believe that they caused the abuse. Adults are responsible for controlling their behavior; children are not.
Children never lie about sexual abuse.	Several court cases have found that children can and do falsely accuse an adult. However, because a child can lie does not mean a child should be ignored. All cases in which a child tells of inappropriate behavior must be investigated thoroughly
There are always physical findings in cases of sexual abuse.	Physical findings, such as the presence of sperm in a child who has not reached puberty, may confirm sexual abuse. In many cases, however, the findings are unclear

46. How should the nurse document findings about suspected abuse or neglect?

All findings should be documented as factually as possible and as completely as possible:
1. Measure all visible symptoms and record the findings in relation to their location.
2. If photographs are taken, the time and authorization for the pictures should be noted. Photographs should be supplemented with accurate written documentation.
3. The exact size and shape of all physical findings should be noted.
4. Chart the parent's comments as exact quotes. For example: "mother states, 'I guess I lost control,'" instead of "mother indicated she may have injured the child."

47. How should the nurse report a potentially abused child?

In the United States and Canada, nurses are required to report all cases in which there is a reasonable suspicion of child abuse. In hospitals, reporting may be handled through the social service department. Reports also may be made through the state or province's protective service agencies or law enforcement agencies. If a nurse is aware of an abusive situation outside the clinical setting, reports can be made anonymously. The nurse never should permit anyone to tell him or her that he or she cannot or should not report a child that the nurse believes is abused. Nurses are protected from liability for reporting child abuse, unless there is indication that a false report was made maliciously.

48. How do nurses deal with their own feelings in cases of child abuse?

The first step is for the nurse to acknowledge his or her own feelings. The nurse may feel a complex set of feelings and emotions on discovering that a child was harmed intentionally. The nurse may experience further frustrations and anger when trying to help the child and family. It is healthy to call in an outside professional to assist the nursing staff in working through their feelings.

CONTROVERSY

49. Discuss the relationship between physical abuse and corporal punishment.

Corporal punishment is the term for using physical pain to control a child's behavior. The exact boundary between corporal punishment and physical abuse is unclear. A spanking on a covered bottom is not considered abusive, whereas leaving permanent damage from punishment is abusive. Many parents and some school districts believe that physical punishment is an appropriate method of controlling child behavior. The Biblical statement of "spare the rod, spoil the child" frequently is cited as justification for corporal punishment and physical abuse. Decreasing the amount of corporal punishment would help to decrease the amount of physical abuse.

BIBLIOGRAPHY

1. Gelles RJ: Intimate Violence in Families, 3rd ed. Thousand Oaks, CA, Sage Publications, 1997.
2. Hansen KK: Folk remedies and child abuse: A review with emphasis on caida de mollera and its relation to shaken baby syndrome. Child Abuse Neglect 22:117–127, 1998.
3. Hayes K, Koziol-McLain J, Johnson M: Abused and neglected patients. In Oman KS, Koziol-McLain J, Scheetz LJ (eds): Emergency Nursing Secrets. Philadelphia, Hanley & Belfus, 2001, pp 235–243.
4. Rickle AU, Becker E: Keeping Children From Harm's Way. Washington, DC, American Psychological Association, 1997.
5. Ripley A: Whippings in the pulpit. Time (April 2):47, 2001.
6. Scales JW, Fleischer AB, Sinal SH, Krowchuk DP: Skin lesions that mimic child abuse. Patient Care 16:169–192, 1999.
7. U.S. Department of Health and Human Services Administration for Children and Families Administration on Children, Youth and Families Children's Bureau: Child Maltreatment 1998: Reports from the States to the National Child Abuse and Neglect Data System. Washington, DC, USDHHS, 1998.
8. Wyszynski ME: Shaken baby syndrome: Identification, intervention, and prevention. Clin Exc Nurse Pract 3:262–267, 1999.

4. THE WELL NEWBORN

Rebecca L. Shabo, RN, CPNP, PhD

1. Define *neonate*.
A human from birth to 28 days of life.

2. Define *infant*.
A human from birth to 1 year of age.

3. What is the Dubowitz score?
A scoring system that uses neurologic and physical characteristics of a newborn that provides an estimate of within 1–2 weeks of gestational age.

4. Why are rales more prominent in the lungs of an infant after birth by cesarean section?
Infants who are born by **cesarean section** do not experience the squeezing of the thorax that is experienced during a vaginal delivery. During this **squeeze**, 30–35 mL of fluid is expelled from the lungs. After birth by cesarean section, rales commonly are heard in the chest for 1 hour before the fluid is reabsorbed.

5. Which bone is broken most commonly during childbirth?
The clavicle.

6. What problem during childbirth most commonly is associated with a broken clavicle?
Shoulder dystocia. The shoulder becomes stuck in the pelvis, and the manipulation needed for delivery often breaks the clavicle.

7. List the signs that may alert the practitioner to the possibility of a fractured clavicle when assessing the newborn.
- Crepitus of the bone
- Limited movement of the affected arm
- No Moro's reflex on the affected side

8. How much weight does an infant lose in the immediate newborn period?
Typically 10% of birth weight.

9. How long does it take for the infant to return to birth weight?
10–14 days.

10. How much weight should a newborn gain after the initial postnatal weight loss?
Approximately 0.5–1 oz/day, or 4–7 oz/week (breast-fed and formula-fed infants).

11. How many hours a day does a newborn typically sleep?
Approximately 16 hours a day, awakening to feed every 1–3 hours.

12. How frequently should a newborn urinate?
6–20 times a day.

13. Why do newborns urinate so frequently?
Renal function is not fully developed until the infant is 2 years old.

14. What is meconium?

The first few stools of the newborn, which contain skin cells, hair, vernix caseosa, blood, mucus, and bile. It is sticky, greenish black, and sometimes difficult to remove from the skin.

15. Are there any tricks for removing meconium from the infant's buttocks?

A dab of zinc oxide (A and D) ointment or petroleum jelly (Vaseline) placed on a wash-cloth is helpful.

16. What are transitional stools?

The stools expected on about the third day of life after the newborn has ingested a suffi-cient amount of milk. They are loose and greenish brown to yellow. They are called **transi-tional stools** because they are transitional between meconium and milk stools, which occur on the fourth day of life.

17. What is a strawberry hemangioma?

A **strawberry** or **superficial hemangioma** is found in the upper dermis of the skin and accounts for most hemangiomas of infancy. These hemangiomas may emerge as a bright red nodule, a pale macule, or a telangiectatic lesion. They typically present at birth or by 4 weeks of age, and involution usually occurs spontaneously between 12 and 15 months of age. Most superficial hemangiomas are flat by 5 years of age.

18. Describe the most common extracranial hemorrhagic head traumas that can occur to newborns during the birth process.

Subgaleal hemorrhage occurs when a force, such as a vacuum, compresses and drags the head through the birth canal. The bleeding extends beyond the bone and continues after birth, putting the infant at risk for serious complications.

Caput succedaneum is an area of edematous tissue and fluid trapped under the scalp but on top of the pericranium. It is caused by the head pressing on the pelvic outlet and typically disappears in about 1 week.

Cephalhematoma is a soft mass of blood trapped beneath the pericranium and confined to one bone. The swelling usually worsens on day 2 or 3 after birth. If there is an absence of skull fracture, the lesion usually resolves in 2 weeks to 3 months.

19. What are Epstein's pearls?

Small epithelial cysts occurring along both sides of the hard palate or along the alveolar ridge. They are not pathologic and disappear with time.

20. Do tear glands function at birth?

No. They typically begin to function at 2–4 weeks of age.

21. What might a high-pitched, shrill cry indicate in a newborn?

Increased intracranial pressure or a condition that affects the central nervous system, such as meningitis.

22. What condition is suggested by absent, weak, or constant crying?

Brain damage.

23. Name a common variation of cardiac rhythm in a newborn.

Sinus arrhythmia (heart rate increases with inspiration and decreases with expiration).

24. Discuss erythema toxicum neonatorum.

Erythema toxicum neonatorum is a pink maculopapular rash that develops in the first few days of life. It resembles varicella or "fleabites." The origin is unknown, and the condi-tion disappears within a few days without treatment.

25. What might tenseness or bulging of the fontanels indicate?

Increased intracranial pressure.

26. In which position should the infant be placed when assessing fontanels for tenseness?

Upright.

27. What is an umbilical granuloma?

Umbilical tissue that sometimes persists after the cord has dried and fallen off. It is sometimes white and glistening, or it may be pink or red.

28. How are umbilical granulomas removed?

By applying silver nitrate.

29. What color of newborn vaginal discharge is considered abnormal?

Yellow discharge could be indicative of infection.

30. List vaginal discharges that are considered normal.

White mucous discharge
A bloody discharge (called **pseudomenstruation**)

31. What causes pseudomenstruation?

Absorption of maternal hormones. This discharge typically stops by 1 month of age.

32. Define oral candidiasis (thrush).

A common disorder of newborns characterized by white patches that adhere to the mouth and tongue.

33. How can these patches be distinguished from coagulated milk?

Thrush cannot be removed with a tongue blade.

34. List the causes of physiologic jaundice in the newborn.

- Higher concentrations of erythrocytes and a shorter life span of red blood cells, producing more **bilirubin** than adults
- Decreased ability of an immature liver to conjugate bilirubin
- Reduced albumin concentrations, which decreases the plasma-binding capabilities for bilirubin

35. Why is breast-feeding associated with an increased risk of physiologic jaundice?

- Decreased fluid intake before milk production may delay hepatic clearance.
- Elements in breast milk, such as fatty acids, may decrease the excretion of bilirubin.

36. What is acrocyanosis?

The **blue color** of the hands and feet during the first few hours to 24 hours after birth.

37. Name the five areas that Apgar scoring assesses.

1. Heart rate
2. Respiratory effort
3. Muscle tone
4. Reflex irritability
5. Color

38. What blood glucose value in a newborn could indicate hypoglycemia?

A heel-stick reading of < 45 mg/100 mL of blood.

39. Why is it important to detect hypoglycemia in a newborn?

The hypoglycemia must be treated quickly because brain damage could result if brain cells are depleted of glucose.

40. List other symptoms of hypoglycemia in a newborn.

Jitteriness
Lethargy
Convulsions

41. Which newborn infants are especially prone to hypoglycemia?

- Low-birth-weight infants (< 2500 g)
- Infants of diabetic mothers
- Infants large for gestational age
- Ill newborns or infants who experienced stress during delivery
- [a] Premature infants (< 37 weeks' gestation)

42. At what age is colic commonly present?

It can begin in the early newborn period and usually decreases or ceases by 3 months of age. Colic episodes generally peak at about **6 weeks**.

43. What is Moro's reflex?

An indicator of neurologic ability in a newborn.

44. How is this reflex tested?

A **Moro**, or **startle, reflex** can be initiated by a loud noise (clapping hands) or quick movement (allow the infant's head to drop back slightly while holding supine). The infant should respond by abducting and extending the arms and legs. The fingers assume a *C* shape.

45. At what age does Moro's reflex disappear?

By the end of the fourth or fifth month.

46. State a typical chest measurement of a newborn in relation to head circumference.

Chest circumference is typically 0.75–1 inch (2 cm) less than head circumference.

47. List four separate mechanisms by which a newborn loses heat.

1. Convection
2. Conduction
3. Radiation
4. Evaporation

48. How can the nurse in the delivery room prevent heat loss through evaporation?

By drying the infant thoroughly of amniotic fluid before giving him or her to the mother.

49. What is cold stress?

The stress that an infant experiences if allowed to become **hypothermic**. There may be decreased oxygen uptake by the lungs, decreased delivery of oxygen to the tissues, and increased anaerobic metabolism.

50. Describe the infant's response to cold stress.

Oxygen and glucose consumption increase, leading to hypoglycemia and hypoxia.

51. Give an example of heat loss through conduction.

Placing an infant on a cold surface, such as a cold scale. Scales should be covered with a warm blanket or heated with a heating lamp before weighing the infant.

52. What is the purpose of the extrusion reflex?

The **extrusion reflex** is a protective reflex that prevents the swallowing of inedible substances. A newborn extrudes substances that are placed on the anterior portion of the tongue. This reflex typically disappears by 4 months of age.

53. Do infants get heartburn?

Infants frequently get **gastroesophageal reflux** during the first year of life. Frequent regurgitation, irritability after feeding, and vomiting may be indicative of this condition. It usually is self-limiting by 6 months to 1 year. In severe cases, failure to thrive, aspiration pneumonia, or esophagitis may be seen. In the preterm infant, gastroesophageal reflux may be associated with apnea.

54. List interventions that can be helpful in managing gastroesophageal reflux in a newborn.
- Small frequent feedings
- Frequent burping during feedings
- Breast-feeding
- Elevate the head of the bed
- Avoid formula changes

55. How should parents be told to dress their infant when they are home?

Dress the child in the same type of clothing that the parent needs to stay comfortable.

56. Name the appropriate size needle to use for the injection of vitamin K and hepatitis vaccine given to the newborn.

25G ⅝-inch needle.

57. What is the preferred site for injection in the newborn?

Vastus lateralis muscle.

BIBLIOGRAPHY

1. Behrman RE: Nelson Textbook of Pediatrics, 15th ed. Philadelphia, W.B. Saunders, 1996.
2. Betz CL, Sowden LA: Pediatric Nursing Reference, 4th ed. St. Louis, Mosby, 2000, pp 170–174.
3. Burns CE, Brady MA, Dunn AM, Starr NB: Pediatric Primary Care: A Handbook for Nurse Practitioners, 2nd ed. Philadelphia, W.B. Saunders, 2000.
4. Frank CG, Cooper SC, Merenstein GB: Jaundice. In Merenstein GB, Gardner SL (eds): Handbook of Neonatal Intensive Care, 4th ed. St. Louis, Mosby, 1998.
5. Glass L: Neonatology. In Finberg L (ed): Saunders Manual of Pediatric Practice. Philadelphia, W.B. Saunders, 1998, pp 46–108.
6. Halamek LP, Stenenson DK: Neonatal hypoglycemia: Pathophysiology and therapy. Clin Pediatr 37:11–16, 1998.
7. Sferra TJ, Heitlinger LA: Gastrointestinal gas formation and infantile colic. Pediatr Clin North Am 43:489–507, 1996.

5. THE HIGH-RISK NEWBORN

Diana Odland Neal, RN, MS

1. What is a high-risk newborn?

A viable infant born between 23 weeks' and 40 weeks' gestation up to 28 days of age after birth, who has a greater than average chance of morbidity or mortality as a result of conditions or events during the prenatal, perinatal, or postnatal periods. Most newborns considered to be at high risk are **preterm** infants (born before the estimated date of delivery).

2. List complications associated with high-risk newborns.

- Respiratory distress
- Hypoglycemia
- Sepsis
- Congenital malformations

3. Describe the Apgar score assigned at delivery of a high-risk newborn.

The Apgar score is made up of five criteria (see Table). All five criteria are evaluated at 1 and 5 minutes after birth and continued every minute until the infant's condition stabilizes. Infants may score up to 2 points per criterion.

Apgar Scoring

ASSESSMENT	0	1	2
Heart rate	Absent	< 100	> 100
Respiratory effort	Absent	Irregular/weak cry	Good/strong cry
Reflex irritability	No response	Grimace	Cough/cry/sneeze
Muscle tone	Flaccid	Some flexion	Spontaneous flexion
Color	Blue/pale	Body pink/extremities blue	Completely pink

4. Discuss respiratory distress.

Respiratory distress is a severe lung disorder and causes the highest infant mortality of any disease. It is a term often used when referring to **respiratory distress syndrome** and **hyaline membrane disease**, which are associated with a developmental delay in the lung maturation of neonates and the absence of surfactant (a substance that reduces the surface tension of the alveoli). Respiratory distress also may be related to **apnea of prematurity** (AOP). It may be a clinical manifestation of nonpulmonary disorders, including hypothermia, cardiac defects such as patent ductus arteriosus (PDA), necrotizing enterocolitis (NEC), intraventricular hemorrhage (IVH), sepsis, and drugs.

5. List elements of assessment for respiratory distress.

Assess the infant for:

Cyanosis	Grunting
Dyspnea	Nasal flaring
Tachypnea	Retractions
Apnea	Low oxygen saturation

6. What are the diagnostic criteria for respiratory distress?

- Arterial blood gas analysis: Pao_2 < 45–60 mmHg; $Paco_2$ > 45–55 mmHg; pH < 7.25–7.35

• Radiographic evaluation: Air bronchograms (**ground-glass** appearance) or patchy infiltrates
• Laboratory specimens (e.g., blood, tracheal aspirates): Positive for white blood cells or various microorganisms

7. **List nursing interventions to support breathing of the high-risk newborn.**
   1. Monitor the infant's respiratory status.
   2. Position the infant.
   3. Keep the airways open and clear of secretions.
   4. Administer medications as ordered.

8. **How is the high-risk newborn's respiratory status monitored?**
   • **Respirations** are monitored through **auscultation** of lung sounds.
   • **Oxygenation** status is monitored through **pulse oximetry, transcutaneous oxygen readings**, and **arterial blood gas analysis**.
   • Episodes of **apnea**, **infant color**, and **self-recovery** or stimulation needed to restore breathing are observed and documented.

9. **What positioning of the high-risk newborn supports breathing?**
   Position the infant in a flexed, side-lying, or prone posture with supportive boundaries and position changes every 2–4 hours. Keep the neck slightly extended with the nose in a "sniffing" position to keep the airway patent.

10. **Describe how an infant should be placed in the prone position.**
   For **prone positioning**, place the infant on top of an infant blanket (folded lengthwise in thirds) with arms and legs flexed around the outside of the blanket in a "crawling posture." Place the infant's hands near the mouth and a pacifier in the mouth if used. Use infant blankets rolled lengthwise as boundaries around the infant to form a **nest** to keep the infant in place.

11. **How is an open airway maintained in a high-risk newborn?**
   For infants with **nasal congestion**, use a bulb syringe to clear nasal passages before feedings and as needed.
   For infants unable to breathe on their own, assist with **endotracheal intubation**. To facilitate the drainage and removal of secretions, provide bronchopulmonary hygiene through chest percussion, vibration, and postural drainage suctioning only as needed to keep airway patent using proper suctioning technique. Position the infant as indicated previously.

12. **What medications may be ordered to support breathing of the high-risk newborn?**
   Medications may be ordered for administration by various routes:
   • Surfactant replacement therapy
   • Nitric oxide
   • Liquid oxygen
   • Nebulizer treatments
   • Caffeine
   • Theophylline
   • Dexamethasone
   • Warmed and humidified supplemental oxygen through:

Oxygen hood	Nasal prongs
Tent	Mechanical ventilation

13. **Describe complications associated with oxygen therapy and mechanical ventilation.**
   • Complications related to **oxygen** therapy include retinopathy of prematurity and bronchopulmonary dysplasia.

• Complications related to **mechanical ventilation** include bronchospasm, hypoxia, IVH, and air leak complications.
• Complications associated with **intubation** include nasal, pharyngeal, or tracheal perforation.

14. Define apnea of prematurity.

A cessation of spontaneous breathing for 20 or more seconds, which may or may not be followed by bradycardia, a change in color, or desaturation. AOP occurs commonly in preterm infants because it is most likely related to **immaturity** of the **respiratory** and **neurologic system**.

15. List the possible causes of neonatal apnea.

• Airway obstruction
• Anemia, hypoxemia, or polycythemia
• Cardiac disorders such as congestive heart failure and PDA
• Central nervous system disorders such as IVH or seizures
• Central nervous system depression from pharmacologic agents
• Dehydration
• Hyperthermia or hypothermia
• Metabolic disturbances such as hypocalcemia, hypoglycemia, and hyponatremia
• NEC
• Sepsis

16. List nursing responsibilities for managing AOP.

1. Observe closely for episodes of apnea and associated bradycardia, color changes, and desaturation.

2. Apply tactile stimulation (gentle rubbing of the feet, chest, or back) or position changes for unrecovered episodes of apnea.

3. Suction the nose and mouth if secretions are present.

4. Administer ordered oxygen for color changes and desaturation.

5. Open the airway and provide positive-pressure ventilation using a bag and mask until breathing is restored.

6. Document the length of apnea, appearance of the infant during and after the apnea spell, and whether the infant self-recovers or requires stimulation to restore breathing.

7. Administer aminophylline, theophylline, or caffeine as ordered to reduce the frequency of apnea spells.

17. What is patent ductus arteriosus?

PDA is a common complication of respiratory distress syndrome in the preterm infant. The ductus remains open after birth of a preterm infant with severe respiratory disease because of the lowered oxygen tension associated with the disease, resulting in left-to-right shunting of blood across the patent ductus.

18. Describe the assessment for PDA.

Clinical manifestations of PDA become apparent within the first week of life. Arterial blood gases for the preterm infant show a decreased Pao_2 and an increased $Paco_2$. The FiO2 is increased, and the infant may exhibit frequent episodes of apnea. The infant may have bounding peripheral pulses, a widening pulse pressure, and a heart murmur. Cardiomegaly is visible on chest radiograph. The diagnosis is confirmed through echocardiography.

19. Discuss the treatment and nursing management for PDA.

Nursing interventions focus on careful cardiovascular and respiratory assessment and close monitoring for complications of therapy. Medical treatment of the PDA using **indomethacin**, a prostaglandin inhibitor used to constrict the ductus, requires close monitoring of the renal system through laboratory analysis of blood urea nitrogen and creatinine and observing for bleeding tendencies or clotting abnormalities. Treatment of the PDA using **surgical ligation** of the ductus necessitates postoperative monitoring for pneumothorax, atelectasis, bleeding, and signs of infection and supportive respiratory care and pain management.

20. Describe the pain experience of infants.

Physiologic responses to pain include flushing, pallor, and diaphoresis of the skin; elevated pulse, respirations, and blood pressure; decreased oxygen saturation; increased muscle tone; dilated pupils; and restlessness.

Behavioral responses to pain include generalized body rigidity, thrashing, crying, and facial expression of pain (brows lowered and drawn together, furrowed forehead, eyes squinting or closed, cheeks raised, nose broadened and bulging, and mouth opened).

Remember, if something is painful to you, it is painful to an infant.

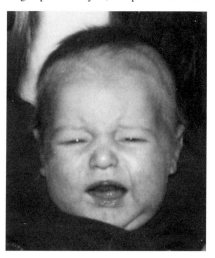

21. Describe the neonatal infant pain scale assessment tool.

Neonatal–Infant Pain Scale (NIPS)

	0	1	2
Facial expression	Relaxed muscles Neutral expression	Tight facial muscles Furrowed brow, chin, jaw	—
Cry	Quiet—not crying	Mild moaning, intermittent cry	Loud scream, rising, shrill, continuous Silent cry (intubated) as evidenced by facial movement
Breathing patterns	Relaxed	Changes in breathing; irregular, faster than usual, gagging, breath holding	—
Arms	Relaxed No muscular rigidity Occasional random movements of arms	Flexed/extended Tense, straight arms, rigid and/or rapid extension, flexion	—

Continued on following page

Neonatal–Infant Pain Scale (NIPS) (continued)

	0	1	2

Legs	Relaxed
	No muscular rigidity
	Occasional random
	  movements of legs
		Flexed/extended
		Tense, straight arms,
		  rigid and/or rapid
		  extension, flexion
			—

State of
  arousal
	Sleeping/awake
	Quiet, peaceful,
	  sleeping, or alert
	  and settled
		Fussy
		Alert, restless, and
		  thrashing
			Constantly awake

From Wong DL, et al: Nursing Care of Infants and Children, 6sth ed. St. Louis, Mosby, 1999, with permission.

22. List nursing interventions for providing comfort to the high-risk newborn.
  1. Administer prescribed opioid analgesics (most commonly morphine)
  2. Provide nonpharmacologic measures individually adjusted in response to infant cues
  Repositioning
  Swaddling
  Cuddling
  Rocking
  Playing soft, soothing music
  Providing gentle touch
  Nonnutritive sucking
  Parents may be encouraged to provide these comfort measures when possible.

23. What is necrotizing enterocolitis?
  NEC is an acute inflammatory disease of the bowel commonly found in high-risk infants. The cause is not known, but the development of NEC is associated with intestinal ischemia, colonization by pathologic bacteria, and formula feeding.

24. Describe the assessment for NEC.
  Clinical manifestations include a distended abdomen, gastric retention, and blood in the stools. The infant may show poor feeding, emesis, decreased urine output, lethargy, apnea, hypothermia, and hypotension.

25. How is NEC diagnosed?
  Radiographic studies show dilation or distention of the bowel and pneumatosis intestinalis (a bubbly appearance of the thickened bowel wall). The radiographic observance of free air in the abdomen indicates perforation of the bowel.
  Laboratory data may indicate anemia, leukopenia, leukocytosis, metabolic acidosis, electrolyte imbalance, and positive blood cultures.

26. Discuss prevention and early recognition of NEC.
  Prevention of NEC is key to its management and consists of delaying oral feedings for infants who are asphyxiated at birth, infants in respiratory distress, and infants born prematurely or of a low birth weight. **Breast milk** is the preferred choice for enteral feedings because of the passive immunity it provides infants.
  Early recognition of NEC consists of measuring residual gastric contents before feedings, auscultation of bowel sounds, and measurement of abdominal girth.

27. List nursing interventions for managing NEC.
  1. Discontinue oral feedings.
  2. Administer intravenous fluids, electrolytes, and antibiotics.

3. Provide oxygen.

4. Maintain gastric decompression per nasogastric suction or gravity drainage.

5. Assist with further diagnostic procedures as ordered.

6. Monitor vital signs.

7. Assess abdominal girth.

8. Wash hands to prevent the spread of infection.

9. Monitor hydration and nutritional management.

10. Reinstitute feedings. Sterile water or electrolyte solution followed by diluted human breast milk or predigested formula is introduced gradually until the infant may tolerate full-strength feedings.

28. Why is adequate hydration of the high-risk preterm infant a challenge?

Extracellular water content is higher, body surface area is greater, and kidneys are immature, increasing the risk of fluid depletion.

29. List nursing interventions for adequate hydration of the high-risk newborn.

1. Monitor the parenteral administration of fluids.

2. Monitor fluid and electrolyte status through:
   • Daily weighing
   • Accurate intake and output of all fluids (including medications, flushes, and blood products)
   • Measurement of urine specific gravity
   • Dipstick urine testing
   • Evaluation of serum electrolytes

3. Prevent complications related to intravenous therapy.

30. How is nutrition provided to high-risk newborns?

Nutrition can be provided parenterally, enterally, or through a combination of the two routes. **Parenteral nutrition** and intravenous lipids routinely are started on the second or third day of life if the infant is metabolically stable. The gradual introduction of **enteral feedings** takes place when the newborn shows adequate oxygenation; thermoregulation; stable cardiovascular status; and evidence of gastrointestinal motility, including feeding tolerance.

31. What forms of enteral nutrition are supplied to high-risk neonates?

Fortified human breast milk is preferred because of the presence of immunoglobulins, leukocytes, lactoferrin, and lysozymes for the added protection against infection. **Premature formulas** are the best substitute.

32. Describe nursing interventions related to feeding the high-risk newborn.

Infants unable to breast-feed or feed from a nipple bottle are provided with continuous drip or intermittent bolus gavage tube feedings until they gain the strength and coordination needed to suck and swallow. Specific nursing interventions include the following:

1. Monitor **parenteral nutrition** carefully and prevent complications related to intravenous therapy.

2. Observe the infant closely for tolerance of **enteral feedings**, noting the amount and characteristics of gastric aspirates, abdominal distention, bowel sounds, stooling patterns, coordination of suck and swallow, respiratory distress, vital signs, and behavioral organization skills (i.e., ability to suck on a pacifier; maintain a quiet, alert state; and engagement cues).

3. Position the infant in a prone or right side-lying position with the head slightly elevated or hold and cuddle the infant in an en face feeding position to promote digestion and to stimulate normal feeding interactions.

4. Provide nonnutritive sucking on a pacifier during gavage feedings and between feedings to promote digestion, oxygenation, oral musculature, and oral stimulation to prevent oral aversion to feedings.

5. Allow for periods of rest between feedings and care procedures to conserve energy for the promotion of growth and development.

33. Why are developmental interventions important for the high-risk newborn?

Developmental interventions are essential to promoting normal growth and development (physiologic and behavioral). The goal is optimal health of the newborn, and all interventions should be individualized for each infant paying close attention to infant cues.

34. How can nurses promote growth and development of the high-risk newborn?

1. Provide **visual stimulation**, such as photographs of parents and siblings, black-and-white objects of various shapes and sizes, and eye contact.

2. Provide **auditory stimulation** of womb sound recordings, soft classical music, soothing parent and sibling voices, and speaking using the infant's name.

3. Provide **olfactory stimulation**, such as breast milk or an article of clothing worn by a parent.

4. Provide **gustatory stimulation** by placing the infant's hand or a pacifier in the mouth or drops of breast milk or formula in the mouth with tube feedings.

5. Provide **tactile stimulation** through gentle touch, stroking, massage, kangarooing (skin-to-skin contact with parent), and a variety of textures.

6. Provide v**estibular stimulation** through an oscillating waterbed, rocking in a chair, range-of-motion exercises, slowly changing position during handling, and grasping of an object.

35. What is intraventricular hemorrhage?

Bleeding into the cavities of the brain. IVH is common in preterm and low-birth-weight infants because of their extensive fragile vascular network of cerebral blood flow. IVH is classified into grades 1 through 4 depending on the degree and severity of the bleeding.

36. Describe the nursing evaluation for IVH.

Grades 1 and 2 IVH may occur without evident clinical manifestations. Signs and symptoms of grades 3 and 4 include an increase in **intracranial pressure** (ICP) resulting in apnea, bradycardia, cyanosis, a full anterior fontanel, increased occipital frontal circumference, separated cranial sutures, anemia, and hypotonia. **Neurologic manifestations** include lethargy, stupor, twitching, and convulsions.

37. How is IVH diagnosed?

Intracranial structures are evaluated through head ultrasonography, computed tomography, or magnetic resonance imaging.

38. List interventions to prevent IVH.

1. Maintain adequate oxygenation.
2. Limit the peak inspiratory pressures on ventilated infants.
3. Avoid acidosis and electrolyte imbalances.
4. Maintain blood pressure within normal limits.
5. Administer isotonic or hypotonic intravenous fluids.
6. Avoid injury through rough handling or overstimulation of high-risk infants.

39. Describe the nursing responsibilities for managing IVH.

Nursing care is focused on **preventing increased ICP** in high-risk neonates. Interventions that may cause injury to these infants must be limited, and interventions aimed at preventing injury, increased blood pressure, and increased ICP must be implemented.

40. List nursing interventions that may cause injury to the high-risk newborn.

NURSING INTERVENTION	INJURY
Environmental stimulation (noise, bright lights, frequent handling)	Increased stress responses ↑ Blood pressure Desaturation ↑ ICP
Nursing care activities (obtaining vital signs, changing diapers, weighing, positioning)	Increased stress responses
Suctioning	Increased blood pressure
Positioning in right side-lying position	Increased ICP
Positioning in poor head-body alignment	Increased ICP

41. How can nurses help prevent injury in the high-risk newborn?

1. Reduce noxious stimulation, such as noise, bright lights, frequent handling, and painful procedures by limiting talk and other noise near the infant, silencing alarms quickly, closing incubator doors quietly, dimming lights, covering incubators with blankets, and providing periods of rest and uninterrupted sleep between care procedures.

2. Handle the high-risk infant slowly and gently during all care procedures.

3. Suction the infant only as needed to keep the airway patent using proper suctioning technique.

4. Position the infant correctly in a flexed left side-lying or prone posture using supportive boundaries and good head-body alignment with the head of the bed elevated 30°.

42. Define sepsis.

The spread of infection from an initial site to the bloodstream resulting in a systemic response also known as **septicemia**. Neonatal sepsis may be acquired prenatally, during delivery, or postnatally.

43. What are some risk factors for neonatal sepsis?

- Neonatal sepsis may be caused by bacterial, viral, fungal, or parasitic **infections**. Neonates have a high risk of septicemia as a result of diminished nonspecific and specific immunity.
- **Preterm** infants are at increased risk because of the premature withdrawal of the placental barrier and interrupted transplacental transmission of immunoglobulins to defend against infection.
- High-risk infants are at increased risk because of **invasive procedures** and **nosocomial exposure** to pathogens in the hospital environment.

44. Discuss the assessment for neonatal sepsis.

Most neonatal infections present with nonspecific, subtle signs and symptoms affecting many different body systems. Nurses may describe the child as "not looking well" or "having a change in behavior." Common clinical manifestations include:

Poor thermoregulation	Poor feeding, emesis, diarrhea, or abdominal distention
Respiratory distress	Lethargy or irritability
Apnea or dyspnea	A full or bulging fontanel
Poor circulation or pallor	Jaundice, ecchymosis, or petechiae

45. How is neonatal sepsis diagnosed?

Definitive diagnosis is made through **laboratory studies** of blood, urine, and cerebrospinal fluid and **radiographic examination**.

46. Describe the nursing management of neonatal sepsis.

Management of the septic infant requires close assessment for clinical manifestations to provide respiratory, circulatory, neurologic, and immunologic support.

Nursing interventions include:
1. Administer oxygen.
2. Provide fluids, electrolytes, and blood transfusions.
3. Observe for seizure activity.
4. Administer antibiotics as ordered.
5. Monitor vital signs.
6. Maintain a neutral thermal environment to prevent hyperthermia or hypothermia.

47. What is hypothermia?

Cold stress that increases oxygen consumption and uses up energy reserves needed for growth and healing processes.

48. Why are preterm and low–birth-weight infants at the greatest risk of hypothermia?

Such infants have less subcutaneous fat and fewer deposits of brown fat for heat production, a larger surface area, smaller muscle mass, and poor reflex control of skin capillaries.

49. What nursing interventions promote thermoregulation in the high-risk newborn?
1. Closely monitor the infant's temperature and regulate the neutral thermal environment.
2. Provide clothing, a head covering, and blanket during removal from the warmer or incubator or skin-to-skin cuddling with parents (kangarooing) when stable.
3. Prevent convective heat loss by reducing air drafts and avoiding blow-by oxygen.
4. Prevent radiant heat loss by using double-walled incubators and avoid placing infants near cold surfaces (e.g., windows, walls).
5. Prevent evaporative heat loss by using a warmed, high-humidity environment. (Change fluids in humidification systems every 8–24 hours to prevent the growth of microorganisms.)
6. Prevent conductive heat loss by warming everything that comes in contact with the infant (e.g., stethoscopes, scales, blankets, hands).

50. List nursing interventions for preventing infection in the high-risk newborn.
1. Wash hands before and after contact with the infant.
2. Clean all equipment and supplies that come in contact with the infant.
3. Prevent visitors and health care workers with communicable illness or infections from having contact with the infant.
4. Isolate infants with communicable illness or infections per agency policy.
5. Ensure that strict medical and surgical asepsis principles are followed by those in contact with the infant.
6. Administer prescribed prophylactic antibiotics and intravenous gamma globulin as ordered.

51. Why is skin care so important in the high-risk newborn?

Maintenance of intact skin is the tiny infant's most effective barrier against infection, insensible fluid loss, protein loss, and blood loss and provides for more effective body temperature control.

52. What nursing interventions promote skin care in the high-risk newborn?
1. Cleanse the oral, diaper, and skin breakdown areas and the eyes daily with plain or sterile warm water when the infant's temperature has stabilized (clean other areas only when needed within the first few weeks of life).
2. Use mild, nonalkaline cleansers as needed for stool removal (avoid soaps and alcohol that dry the skin).

3. Apply moisturizing agents after bathing to retain moisture and rehydrate the skin (clean off old creams and ointments before applying a new layer).

4. Use topical agents that may be absorbed into the skin sparingly and only when necessary (e.g., adhesive removers, hydrogen peroxide, tincture of benzoin).

5. Use minimal tape and adhesives, and use protective skin barriers where tape and adhesives are used (i.e., for securing endotracheal tubes, gavage tubes, temperature probes).

6. Prevent pressure areas by using pressure-reducing mattresses or sheepskin and frequent position changes.

7. Protect bony prominences, such as knees and elbows, with skin barriers (Tegaderm) as needed to prevent skin breakdown.

8. Closely monitor the use of warm packs, heating pads (Aqua-K pads), or other heating devices, and avoid the use of heat lamps and transcutaneous electrodes whenever possible (use pulse oximetry instead of transcutaneous monitoring on preterm and low-birth-weight infants).

9. Secure intravenous catheters with commercial intravenous protectors with minimal tape and maximal visualization of the fingers, toes, and intravenous site.

10. Document the condition of the skin and skin care provided.

53. Define neonatal abstinence syndrome.

This term describes the signs of drug withdrawal exhibited by infants exposed to chemical substances in utero.

54. How is neonatal abstinence syndrome assessed?

The clinical manifestations of **neonatal abstinence syndrome** depend on the amount, type, and length of time the maternal chemical was used and the drug level at the time of delivery. Signs and symptoms may appear 3 weeks or more after birth and may persist for 3–4 months. Some infants of **heroin**-addicted mothers may not show signs of withdrawal, and infants of **cocaine**-addicted mothers may exhibit lethargy, hypotonia, decreased birth weight, and decreased length.

55. List common signs of withdrawal in neonatal abstinence syndrome.

Irritability	Poor feeding
Restlessness	Frantic sucking of the fists between feedings
Hyperactivity	Vomiting
Increased muscle tone	Diarrhea
Tremors	Temperature instability
Sweating	Tachypnea
High-pitched and shrill cry	Frequent sneezing
Insomnia	Excoriation of the knees, nose, cheeks, and toes
Frequent yawning	

56. Describe the nursing management of neonatal abstinence syndrome.

Nursing care of drug-exposed infants is directed toward **reducing noxious stimuli**, such as noise, bright lights, frequent handling, and painful procedures by limiting talk and other noise near the infant, silencing alarms quickly, closing incubator doors quietly, dimming lights, covering incubators with blankets, and providing periods of rest and uninterrupted sleep between care procedures.

Other nursing interventions include the provision of adequate fluids and nutrition, monitoring of intake and output, snug swaddling in a blanket, rocking, and the prevention of skin abrasions through skin barriers such as Tegaderm on the knees, nose, cheeks, and toes.

Careful **documentation** of clinical manifestations assists in evaluating the severity of the infant's withdrawal symptoms and the pharmacologic management needed.

Supportive care and referral to community social services of the often anxious, depressed, and defensive mother is vital if she is to resume responsibility for care of her infant after discharge from the hospital.

57. Why is the birth of a high-risk newborn a stressful event for parents?

Parents are anxious about the viability and normalcy of their infant. They are overwhelmed with feelings of responsibility, expense, and frustration as they often are faced with multiple crises coping with their own needs, the needs of their infant, and the needs of other family members.

58. What nursing interventions can help support families of a high-risk newborn?

1. Provide parents with information about the infant's status and progress and involve them in patient care conferences with other health care providers.

2. Encourage the family to ask questions and verbalize concerns about the infant.

3. Be honest, caring, and sensitive in responding to questions and emphasize positive aspects of the infant's behavior and development.

4. Encourage family visits (parents, grandparents, and siblings) and calls and involvement in caring for and comforting the infant.

5. Show and assist parents with infant care techniques and developmental interventions and help them to understand and respond to infant cues.

6. Refer family members to appropriate agencies, services, and support groups as needed.

BIBLIOGRAPHY

1. Beachy P, Beacon J: Core Curriculum for Neonatal Intensive Care Nursing. Philadelphia, W.B. Saunders, 1999.
2. Furdon SA, Pfeil VC, Snow K: Operationalizing Donna Wong's principle of atraumatic care: Pain management protocol in the NICU. Pediatr Nurs 24:336–342, 1998
3. Gomella TL, et al: Management of low birth weight infants during the first week of life. In Neonatology: Management, Procedures, On-Call Problems, Diseases and Drugs, 4th ed. Stamford, CT, Appleton & Lange, 1999, pp 113–124.
4. Theobald K, Botwinski C, Albanna S: Apnea of prematurity: Diagnosis, implications for care, and pharmacological management. Neonatal Network 19:17–26, 2000.
5. Wong DL, Hockenberry-Eaton M, Wilson D: Nursing Care of Infants and Children, 6th ed. St. Louis, Mosby, 1999.

6. BREAST-FEEDING

Patricia M. Murphy, RNC, MSN, IBCLC,
and Kathleen M. Moonan, RNC, M., IBCLC

1. Should every mother breast-feed?

This is an individual decision for each woman to make. It is the health care professional's responsibility to inform the expectant mother adequately about the benefits of breast-feeding and to provide opportunities for her to make an informed decision. There should be no guilt associated with the decision to use artificial feedings, but the practitioner should ascertain that the woman is making an informed choice. The expectant woman should be aware of any contraindications to breast-feeding.

2. What are the benefits of breast milk for the infant?

Breast milk is suited perfectly to the human infant. It is readily available and easily digested, the composition changing during a feed and with the age of the infant. Breast milk contains **long-chain polyunsaturated fatty acids** essential for development of the neurologic system in the first year of life. Individuals fed breast milk the first 6 months of life have IQs on average 8–12 points higher than other individuals. **Secretory immunoglobulin A (IgA)** is the major antibody in human milk and causes lower incidence of gastrointestinal and upper respiratory infections. Other benefits include decreased incidence of necrotizing enterocolitis, ulcerative colitis, Crohn's disease, sudden infant death syndrome, and childhood cancers and a reduced risk of insulin-dependent diabetes mellitus.

3. List the benefits of breast-feeding for the mother.
- Decreased postpartum hemorrhage
- Increased weight loss postpartum
- Decreased risk of premenopausal breast cancer
- Decreased risk of ovarian cancer
- Decreased osteoporosis
- Lactation amenorrhea
- Later return of fertility
- Increased maternal–infant bonding

4. Are there other benefits to breast-feeding?

Yes. In general, breast-feeding benefits society through:
- Decreased health care costs
- Increased productivity in the workplace
- Decreased absenteeism
- Significant reduction in infant morbidity and mortality
- No usage of land resources or chemicals that add to pollution
- No waste added environmentally

5. Why it is important to initiate breast-feeding within the first hour after birth?

Early initiation of breast-feeding is associated with breast-feeding success. If the infant is exposed to the breast soon after birth, he or she becomes familiar with the mother's scent and the feel of her skin and is able to latch on more effectively. If the infant does not breast-feed soon after birth, he or she goes into a deep sleep and may not awaken for a feed. Hospital policies may direct the staff to give other fluids to the infant, introducing artificial feeds unnecessarily. Infants at risk need to orient to the breast early rather than be introduced to bottles that may interfere with breast-feeding success.

6. Describe proper positioning of the infant at the breast.

The mother needs to be in a comfortable position. The infant needs to be placed at the level of the breast, facing the mother and aligned so that when the infant's mouth is open wide, he or she can be brought well onto the breast. Proper alignment includes supporting the infant at the base of the neck but not forcing the back of the head. Looking down at the infant, the ear, shoulder, and spine should be in alignment. If positioned across the mother, the infant should be tummy-to-tummy with the mother. The mother needs to support her breast like a *C* to keep the infant from slipping down and causing damage to the nipple.

7. Describe the three most common positions.

1. **Cross cradle.** The mother supports the infant with her forearm, with her hand open and supporting the base of the infant's head. The infant's body faces the mother. Her free hand supports the breast in a *C* hold. This gives her more control to bring the infant onto the breast successfully. (See Figure on following page.)

2. **Side-lying.** The mother lies on her side in bed, with her breast resting on the mattress, and brings the infant onto the breast. The infant lies on his or her side facing the mother. This position is recommended after a difficult vaginal delivery.

3. **Side football or clutch.** The mother holds the infant along the side that she plans to breast-feed. The infant's body is held with the mother's arm supporting the back and neck, facing the mother's body. The infant can be wrapped around her side or in a semi-seated position facing the mother's breast.

8. What are the four A's of assessing the infant at the breast?

Alignment
Areolar grasp
Areolar compression
Audible swallow[11]

9. How can you determine an effective latch at the breast?

1. Are the infant's lips flanged out?
2. Are cheeks full?
3. Do you see long extension of the chin well into the breast?
4. Are the sucks fast or becoming rhythmic?
5. Does the mother say it hurts less within the first minute?

10. Explain the difference between a nutritive and nonnutritive suck.

A **nutritive suck** at the breast consists of a rhythmic suck, audible swallow, and breathing pattern that usually lasts approximately 15 minutes or more. The infant who is sucking correctly slows down at the end of the feeding at the breast and often comes off on his or her own, seeming satiated.

A **nonnutritive suck** is one that remains rapid; the infant does not switch to long, rhythmic suck and swallow; and when removed, the infant is not satiated.

11. How can you tell if a breast-fed infant is adequately hydrated?

1. Is the infant nursing at least 8–12 times a day?
2. Is the infant nursing at least 15–20 minutes on one or both breasts every 2–3 hours?
3. Is the infant wetting 6–8 diapers per day at 1 week of age?
4. Is the infant stooling at least 4 times per 24 hours?
5. Have the stools changed color and consistency from the black meconium to a loose, seedy, yellow brownish stool?
6. Is the infant gaining at least 0.5–1 oz of weight per day?
7. Does the infant seem satiated after a feeding?
8. Do the mother's breasts feel less full after the feeding?

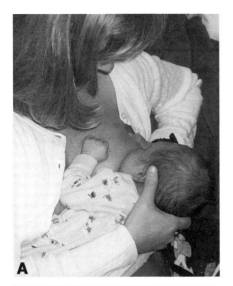

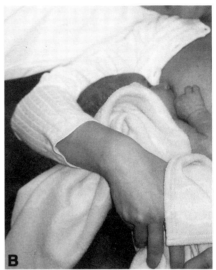

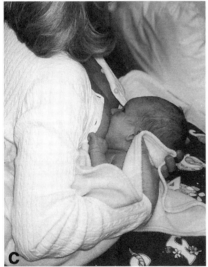

The three most common breast-feeding positions.
A, Cross-cradle position. *B*, Side-lying position.
C, Side football or clutch position.

12. What should breast-feeding mothers know about feeding frequency and duration?

- The newborn needs to feed at least 8–12 times in 24 hours. That averages out to about every 2–3 hours.
- The infant should maintain a rhythmic suck and audible swallow for about 15–20 minutes on the first breast and probably will do about the same at the second breast. The mother needs to be reassured that the newborn may only take one breast at a feeding and awaken in 1–1.5 hours to feed on the second breast.
- It is important to teach the mother to watch the infant feed, not the clock.

13. Is supplemental water necessary in the breast-feeding infant?

No. As long as the infant is feeding correctly and gaining weight, no extra water is needed. Breast milk is composed of 87% water; if a mother is concerned about fluids, she should increase breast-feeding sessions.

14. How does supplementation affect breast-feeding?

The easiest way to instruct parents about the hazards of supplementation is to review the supply and demand principle. If the infant is nursing regularly or the mother is pumping her breasts at regular intervals, the brain receives the message to release oxytocin and prolactin, the hormones responsible for releasing the milk and producing more milk. If the mother supplements and the breasts are not stimulated by the infant nursing or pumping, the brain gets no stimulus to release more hormones. Thus, if supplementation becomes more frequent or bottles are given at regular feeding times, the milk supply decreases.

15. What is cluster feeding?

A term given to the frequent feeds an infant demands in the early days of life, usually at a given time of day (most frequently at night when the parents are ready for a night's sleep). The infant may feed for 20 minutes on each breast, fall asleep, and awaken to feed again. Cluster feeding can occur for a 4- to 6-hour stretch of close feedings.

16. How can the nurse help a mother through the cluster feeding period?

Because the mother will be exhausted, she needs to be reassured that cluster feeding is usually associated with the early establishment of her milk supply and the cluster feeding pattern should cease after several days. The mother needs to be well nourished and hydrated. The mother needs to be relaxed, to keep the infant skin-to-skin, and to continue feeding the infant as needed. The mother and infant should be assessed for correct positioning, correct suck and swallow, and adequate transfer of breast milk.

17. During the early weeks of breast-feeding, what factors interfere with breast-feeding success?

Early introduction of **formula** and bottles is the most destructive factor. Early **separation** of the mother and infant also contributes.

18. Describe the normal voiding and stooling pattern of the breast-feeding infant in the early weeks of life.

By the end of the first week of life, the infant needs to wet 6–8 diapers/24 hours and stool at least 4–12 times/24 hours. Often, the newborn stools more than wets when the mother's milk has been established.

19. What instructions should breast-feeding mothers be given at discharge?

Prior to discharge, a breast-feeding mother should be instructed:
- To make sure the is infant feeding at least 8–12 times in 24 hours
- To check that the infant is latched on correctly
- To check that the infant is transferring milk
- To make sure the infant is wetting, stooling, and gaining weight
- To keep phone numbers of community resources available to provide accurate breast-feeding counseling

20. Describe the normal weight gain pattern of the breast-fed infant.

The breast-feeding newborn typically loses weight in the first 3–4 days of life (7–10%). When the mother's milk supply is established, the breast-feeding newborn gains about 1 oz/day. The preferred weight gain in the breast-feeding infant is 1–2 oz/day, although many health care providers accept a gain of 0.5–1 oz/day for the first 6 months of life.

21. What is the recommended treatment for sore nipples in the breast-feeding mother?

- Assess nipple damage.
- Assess for correct latch, rhythmic suck, and audible swallow during feeding.
- Apply moist heat and massage the breast before a feeding to facilitate the let-down reflex, reducing the infant's rapid suckling.

• Initiate feedings on the least sore side.
• After feeding, express some colostrum and air dry the nipple.
• Depending on the nipple damage, it may be necessary to use an antibiotic ointment topically or a purified lanolin.
• A **hydrogel disk** can be applied topically to alleviate nipple pain and facilitate healing.
• Hard, plastic breast shells have been used to reduce friction from fabric and to aid in healing the breast.

22. Discuss the use of nipple shields.
Research supports use of a silicone breast shield to keep the infant at the breast and reduce nipple trauma. If the mother is using a nipple shield, it is imperative to monitor the infant's output to ensure the milk flow is adequate. Use of a **hospital-grade breast pump** may be indicated to increase milk supply while using a nipple shield.

23. When is use of a nipple shield indicated?
• Sore, cracked, bleeding nipples (when the mother is ready to quit breast-feeding)
• Latching difficulties or sucking concerns
• Assisting a preterm infant to the breast
• Infant refusal of the breast
• Overactive let-down of milk

24. What is breast engorgement?
The breast fills with milk approximately 3 days after delivery. Blood supply to this area increases as lactogenesis begins. As the milk glands and ducts fill up, the surrounding tissue becomes fuller and congested. The breast is shiny and taut, and mothers may complain of discomfort. As the breast gets fuller, an everted nipple becomes flatter, making it difficult for the infant to latch.

25. How is breast engorgement treated?
• Frequent emptying of the breast, avoiding supplementation
• Heat and massage before latch to facilitate let-down reflex
• Cool packs after feedings

26. What if these treatments don't work and engorgement becomes severe?
Cool green cabbage leaves can be applied to the breast to reduce swelling and to increase milk flow. The cabbage leaves must be layered around the breast and left on until they wilt. The mother can repeat this once or twice during the engorgement period, but frequent applications may affect milk supply. Cabbage leaves are thought to contain a substance similar to that found in sulfa drugs. If a mother is allergic to sulfa drugs, she is cautioned against the use of cabbage leaves.

27. What is a plugged duct?
A blockage within a milk duct, which is caused by poor positioning of the infant at the breast, inadequate emptying of the breast, missed feedings, engorgement, or external pressure on the breast.

28. How is a plugged duct treated?
• Frequent emptying of the breast
• Use of heat and massage to unplug the blockage
• Alternate positions of the infant at breast to empty the breast better
The mother should use a larger nursing bra or bra extender. She should avoid the use of underwire bras and pulling the bra up to breast-feed. This adds pressure to the breast.

29. What is thrush?
Oral candidiasis, a yeastlike fungal infection. Women who have been taking antibiotics often are more prone to the development of thrush. Candidiasis can present as a vaginal infection,

with thick white discharge. If the infant is exposed during delivery, he or she can develop **oral thrush**. The infant with oral thrush can pass it to the mother through breast-feeding. The infant may not seem bothered but usually has white patches on the gums, tongue, and lining of the oral mucosa. The mother complains of sharp burning pain in the nipple and often into the breast. The pain is associated not only with latching on, but often also during and after the feeding.

30. How is thrush treated?
- Oral **nystatin** is swabbed on infant's oral mucosa, gums, and tongue after a feeding.
- The mother needs to adhere to careful hand washing, using paper towels to dry hands.
- The mother can apply a **topical agent** (usually miconazole, clotrimazole, or nystatin) to nipples after rinsing with a vinegar and water solution. Before feeding, the mother should rinse off any residual ointment that remains on the nipple.
- In **resistant cases, gentian violet** (0.25–1%) solution can be applied to the infant's mouth and mother's nipples twice a day for 3 days.
- For **ductal candidiasis**, the mother should be given oral **fluconazole**.

It is important to counsel the mother about household cleaning during a yeast outbreak and to advise her to take acidophilus, garlic, zinc, and B vitamins to boost her immune system. She should reduce her intake of sugar and dairy products during a yeast outbreak.

31. What is mastitis?
An infection in the breast. It is commonly seen after 10 days postpartum, with the highest incidence between the second and third week. It is usually unilateral but can be bilateral with a sudden onset. The breast-feeding mother complains of localized breast pain or a red, hot, swollen lump; an elevated temperature; and flulike symptoms. Mastitis is associated with *Staphylococcus aureus* and occasionally *Streptococcus*.[6]

32. What factors predispose for mastitis?
Poor or infrequent drainage of the breast
Cracked or fissured nipples
Fatigue and stress

33. How is mastitis treated?
- Mastitis is treated best with frequent emptying of the involved breast, moist heat to the area before and during feeding, and massage to the affected breast before and during feeding.
- The mother should increase fluids, increase rest, and decrease stress.
- Antibiotics are prescribed for 10–14 days. The standard antibiotic is **penicillinase-resistant penicillin** or **cephalosporin**.
- It is important to educate the mother regarding signs and symptoms of yeast infections that may occur secondary to antibiotic therapy.[6]

34. What is a white bleb on the nipple of a breast-feeding mother?
This often is described by the mother as a **white dot**. The **white bleb** appears on the surface of the nipple, frequently at the opening of the duct. It measures ≤ 1 mm in diameter and is shiny and smooth. Breast-feeding mothers complain of extreme pain while feeding.[6]

35. How is a white bleb treated?
If the infant's suckling does not clear the bleb, application of warm compresses before feeding may open the duct. Treatment frequently is done by a health care professional with a sterile needle. The bleb may reappear and require further treatment because it sometimes is caused by yeast.

36. Discuss galactoceles.
Galactoceles are milk-filled cysts. They occur infrequently and are found most commonly in the breast-feeding mother. Galactoceles can predispose the mother to plugged ducts,

mastitis, and breast abscess. No single treatment has been effective. Aspiration has been used; however the lump may refill. A galactocele can be removed surgically under local anesthesia. Regardless of the treatment, breast-feeding should not be interrupted.[6]

37. What is a breast abscess?

An accumulation of pus in the breast tissue. A small percentage of breast-feeding mothers with mastitis develop a breast abscess.[6]

38. How is a breast abscess treated?

Treatment depends on the size of the abscess. If it is small on ultrasound scan, it is **aspirated** with a fine needle. **Incision and drainage** by a physician is recommended for larger abscesses. Treatment also includes frequent emptying of the breast, increased rest, warm soaks, and appropriate antibiotic therapy.[6]

39. Can a mother continue to breast-feed with a breast abscess?

Yes. Unless the abscess opens into the ductal system, the milk is safe for breast-feeding. Complete emptying of the breasts every few hours is part of the treatment. Breast-feeding is encouraged as long as the incision and drainage tube is far from the areola and not involved in the feeding.

40. What if the mother is unable to breast-feed or chooses not to?

The breast should be drained manually to maintain the milk supply. Breast-feeding can resume when sufficient healing has occurred, usually in approximately 4 days. During the treatment and healing, the infant can continue to feed on the unaffected side.

41. Discuss the impact of maternal illness on breast-feeding.

Any acute or chronic maternal health problem may affect lactation significantly. The physical and emotional health of the mother has a direct impact on her ability to provide care for her infant. If the mother is experiencing a serious health condition, she and her infant must be monitored closely by a health care provider. Only in unusual circumstances is it advised that the mother not breast-feed. The benefits of breast-feeding almost always outweigh the risks of not breast-feeding.

42. Can a mother with hepatitis B virus breast-feed?

Yes. The infant should be given hepatitis B immunoglobulin within 12 hours after birth. After the initial immunization, the infant should be given a series of three injections of hepatitis B virus vaccine at 1 week, 1 month, and 6 months. The infant should be monitored by a health care provider.

43. How does breast surgery affect breast-feeding?

The woman's ability to breast-feed depends on:
• The type of surgery
• The surgical technique
• Intactness of neural pathways and blood supply
• The amount of tissue removed

The two most common types of breast surgery performed in women of childbearing age are breast reduction and breast augmentation.

1. **Breast reduction** frequently is done to decrease discomfort from neck and back pain. The ability to breast-feed depends on whether nerve pathways are functional, whether the blood supply remains intact, and how much tissue is removed. Breast-feeding is possible in instances in which the nipple and areola remain attached and a wedge of tissue is removed from the breast. In this type of procedure, the breast ducts, nerve pathways, and blood supply remain intact.

2. **Breast augmentation** frequently is done for cosmetic reasons. The four different types of augmentation surgery vary primarily in the location of the surgical incision. With the exception of the transareolar technique, augmentation frequently has little impact on the initial success of breast-feeding. Women who have augmentation surgery often fear silicone leakage into the breast milk and increased risk of breast cancer. Pressure from the implants also can cause diminished milk production.

Women who have had breast surgery may not be able to breast-feed exclusively. These women need the best possible follow-up after discharge from the hospital. The infant must have frequent assessments for adequate intake and weight gain.[6]

44. What can be done if the infant is not getting enough milk from the breast?
A lactation aid may be useful to provide necessary supplementation.
Medications and herbal remedies may help to increase the mother's milk supply.

45. Can a breast-feeding mother take prescription medications?
Most medications are safe to take during breast-feeding. Some of the significant information to be considered when prescribing medication for breast-feeding mothers includes:

Adult half-life   Plasma peak   Oral bioavailability
Pediatric half-life   Protein binding   Molecular weight[4]
Milk-to-plasma ratio

46. When is breast-feeding contraindicated?
- Untreated active pulmonary tuberculosis
- Human immunodeficiency virus (HIV)
- Human T-cell leukemia virus
- Maternal substance abuse
- Current chemotherapy treatment
- Radiopharmaceuticals
- Maternal galactosemia
- Active herpes lesion on the nipple

47. Is breast-feeding still contraindicated when herpes lesions on the nipple have healed?
No.

48. What signs indicate insufficient milk supply to the infant?
- Fewer than 6 wet diapers or 4 stools in a 24-hour period
- Fewer than 7 breast-feeding sessions per day
- Greater than 10% loss of body weight
- Long nighttime periods without feeding
- Infant not satisfied after a feeding
- Infant does not wake for feedings
- Infant shows signs of dehydration:
  Dry mucous membranes
  Uric acid crystals in the diaper
  Skin tenting
- Long breast-feeding sessions, with rapid suckling and few swallows
- Breasts softer, less sensation of let-down, or no leaking of breast milk
- Introduction of frequent artificial feedings

49. Can the mother increase her milk supply?
Yes. The mother's ability to increase her milk supply depends on (1) the age of the infant, (2) the infant's ability to latch and breast-feed correctly, and (3) the glandular activity in the mother's breasts. The following may help increase milk supply:

- Accurate assessment of the infant's latch and effective suckling
- Increased frequency and duration of breast-feeding during the day and at night
- Use of both breasts at a feeding to increase stimulation
- Skin-to-skin contact
- The use a hospital-grade pump to provide additional stimulation to the breasts
- Balanced maternal diet with adequate hydration, B vitamins, use of **galactagogues** (food, drinks, herbs)
- Rest and relaxation

50. Is there a specific diet for the breast-feeding mother?

No. The breast-feeding mother should eat a nutritious diet based on the U.S. Department of Agriculture's food guide pyramid groups. The breast-feeding mother should increase her total number of calories per day to 2200.

51. Give an example of an adequate diet for the breast-feeding mother.

FOOD GROUP	DAILY INTAKE
Milk or milk products	3 servings
Meat or meat substitute	7 oz
Eggs	1–2 servings
Fruit	3–4 servings
Vegetables	4–5 servings
Grains	9–11 servings

52. How much fluid should a lactating woman consume each day?

To ensure adequate hydration, she should have 8 or more cups of fluid each day. Most women consume this through their natural sense of thirst, but women can remind themselves to meet this need by drinking something every time they feed the infant.

53. What are galactagogues?

Foods, medications, or herbs that are thought to have properties that increase the amount of a mother's milk supply. Dietary galactagogues vary among cultures. Cultures differ in the foods that are encouraged and the foods that are restricted.

54. Discuss the use of herbs as galactagogues.

Although there is there is little scientific research to support their use, anecdotal evidence seems to support the use of herbs in some situations, if used as directed. Two herbs found to be useful in increasing milk supply are **fenugreek** and **blessed thistle**. They are available in tea and capsule form. Teas are not always as effective because of the large amount of tea that needs to be consumed. Other herbs available include fennel, goat's rue, and garlic.

55. Are any prescription medications promoted as galactagogues?

Metoclopramide (Reglan) is a prescribed medication that increases breast milk volume by stimulating prolactin release and blocking dopamine. It is available in tablet form. Women frequently notice an improvement in the milk supply in approximately 3 days. Side effects need to be discussed with the provider. This medication is not recommended for women treated for anxiety, agitation, or depression.

56. Does the breast-feeding mother require dietary supplements to produce adequate milk?

No, if the mother understands and follows the guidelines presented by the food guide pyramid.

57. What are alternative feeding practices?

Feeding practices that avoid the use of artificial nipples to provide nutrition to a breast-feeding infant ($\geq$ 32 weeks' gestation). The options available for alternative feeding include cup feeding, a tube feeding device used at the breast, and a tube feeding device used for finger feeding.

58. When are alternative feeding practices indicated?

When a mother's milk supply is low, an infant is unable to latch onto the breast, or an infant is sick and requires supplemental nutrition, the following practices may be tried.

1. **Finger feeding** is indicated when:
   • The infant is not able to establish a sucking pattern and suck training is required
   • The mother is unable to nurse the infant at the breast because of maternal-infant separation or the mother's nipples are damaged
   • The infant is more than 24 hours old and has not latched successfully
   • The infant is not removing the milk from the breast effectively and requires supplementation after a feeding
2. A t**ube-feeding device** at the breast is indicated when:
   • The infant has a weak suck or tires easily and requires a supplement (the supplement can be given during the feeding)
   • The mother has a low milk supply and the infant requires a supplement
3. **Cup feeding** is indicated when:
   • The infant is separated from the mother
   • The mother is unable to nurse the infant at the breast
   • The infant is not able to latch on for the feeding
   • The infant has a weak suck and is not able to latch or finger feed
   • The infant is not using the tongue correctly (cup feeding helps to bring the tongue down and past the gum lines)

59. Define colic.

Extreme fussiness in the infant. The infant who is experiencing colic often has a piercing cry and severe abdominal discomfort and cannot be comforted. The infant appears to suffer from extreme discomfort most of the time, typically following a feeding.[5]

60. What causes colic?

The exact cause is unknown. Some theories relate colic to **stress and tension** in the mother and infant. Others believe the cause is related to **immature digestive and intestinal system** or **allergies**. Approximately 16–30% of all infants experience colic symptoms. In most infants, colic symptoms disappear by 16 weeks of age.[5]

61. Are breast-fed infants more likely to develop colic than bottle-fed infants?

No. Colic is seen less frequently in breast-fed infants.

62. Discuss breast-feeding and returning to work.

Returning to work and continuing to breast-feed is a challenge. Several things can help ease the transition:

1. During the maternity leave, the mother should establish a good milk supply. The mother should rent or purchase a breast pump that is convenient, high quality (ideally a hospital-grade or professional-grade pump), and accommodates a double pump kit. The mother should initiate a regular pumping schedule to increase her milk supply and to begin collecting milk for storage.

2. Between 3 and 6 weeks, the mother should introduce a bottle to the infant so that the infant becomes receptive to it.

3. The mother should empty her breasts at least every 3 hours while away from infant.

4. During the evenings, nights, and weekends, the mother should breast-feed as often as possible.

5. The mother should contact her employer before returning to work to determine if the company sponsors support for breast-feeding mothers.

63. How does a mother choose an appropriate breast pump?

A mother should base her breast pump selection on her pumping needs and financial ability. There are four types of pumps:

1. **Hospital-grade pumps** are the most expensive type. They are designed for double or single pumping, are heavy in weight, and allow for adjustable speed and suction. They are ideal for a mother with a premature or sick infant. Examples include the Medela Classic (Medela, Inc., McHenry, IL), Medela Lactina Select, and Hollister-Egnell (Hollister Ameda Egnell, Libertyville, IL).

2. **Professional-grade pumps** are more affordable than hospital-grade pumps. They are efficient, durable, and lightweight; they allow for single or double pumping; and they have adjustable speed and suction. They are excellent for a mother who is returning to work and needs to pump 3–4 times daily. Examples include Medela Pump in Style and Hollister-Egnell Purely Yours.

3. **Small electric pumps** are intended for mothers who do not pump frequently. They are not as efficient or durable as professional or hospital-grade pumps. Examples include Medela Mini Electric and Nurture III.

4. **Manual pumps** operate through a hand-held single pump or through hand expression by the mother. Manual pumps vary in price, efficiency, and durability. Examples include Egnell On-Hand Breast Pump, Medela Spring Express, and the Avent "Isis" pump (Avent America, Inc., Bensenville, IL).

64. If a mother is pumping and feeding expressed breast milk in a bottle, how does she estimate the amount of fluid needed per feeding?

A simple calculation is to take the infant's weight in pounds and multiply it by 2.5. This gives an estimate of the total ounces of fluid required in 24 hours. Divide this amount by 8 (estimate of feeds per 24 hours) to give an approximate amount to prepare per feed.

Example: For an infant weighing 10 lb: $2.5 \times 10 = 25$ oz/day; $25 \div 8 \cong 3$ oz per feed.

65. How should expressed breast milk be stored?

• Freshly expressed breast milk can remain at **room temperature** for approximately 10 hours.
• Breast milk can be **refrigerated** for 5–7 days.
• Breast milk can be stored in a **self-contained freezer** unit of a refrigerator for 3–4 months.
• Breast milk can be stored in a **deep freezer** at 0°F for 6 months to 1 year.
• Breast milk can be frozen in glass containers, clear hard plastic containers, and plastic bags designed for breast milk storage.

66. Can expressed breast milk be combined with previously expressed breast milk?

• When both breasts are pumped at the same feeding, the bottles can be combined for storage.
• Chilled milk from multiple pumping sessions can be combined for storage if collected in close proximity. The milk should be labeled with the date and time of the earliest pumping.
• Newly pumped milk can be added to previously frozen milk after it has chilled 2 hours. To prevent the frozen milk from partially defrosting, the amount of newly added milk should be less than the frozen. The milk should be labeled with the date and time of the earliest pumping.

67. Describe the appropriate methods for defrosting and warming human milk.

1. Milk may be thawed by placing it in the refrigerator for 24 hours. After 24 hours, if it is not used, the milk must be discarded. It cannot be refrozen.

2. Milk can be thawed in a pan of warm water or under a stream of warm tap water. The milk should be used within 24 hours.

Microwave ovens should *not* be used to thaw breast milk. Microwave ovens create hot spots that can burn the infant's mouth. Microwaving also has been found to decrease activity of anti-infective properties.

68. What is ankyloglossia?

A tight frenulum, a defect in the infant's mouth. The membrane is too short and limits the tongue's movement.[5]

69. What is the impact of ankyloglossia on breast-feeding?

The infant is unable to move the tongue forward enough to grasp the nipple and areola sufficiently. If the infant is able to latch, the mother initially complains of nipple soreness throughout the feeding, caused by inappropriate suckling. Nipple soreness is followed by poor weight gain in the infant and a possible a decrease in the mother's milk supply.

70. How is ankyloglossia treated?

The lingual frenulum can be clipped by a qualified health care professional. Mothers frequently note a relief from nipple pain and a change in the infant's suckling pattern. In some instances, clipping is not necessary. The frenulum over time is stretched by the suckling action. The severity of maternal and infant conditions determines the interventions.

71. Discuss tandem nursing.

Tandem nursing is breast-feeding more than one sibling of different ages. If the mother chooses to breast-feed while pregnant, she must be sure to consume enough nutrients to meet her own nutritional needs, the needs of the growing fetus, and the needs of the older child. If the mother continues to breast-feed more than one infant after birth, milk supply is not an issue. The increased feeding creates a supply for the older child and infant. To ensure that the infant gets enough milk, the mother should breast-feed the infant first, or the mother can breast-feed the same child on the same breast, switching daily.

72. What birth control options are available for the breast-feeding mother?

Tubal ligation
Lactational amenorrhea (barrier
    devices suggested)
Natural family planning
Nonprescription methods:
  Foam   Jellies
  Condoms   Creams

Prescription methods:
  Oral contraceptive
  Injectable medroxyprogesterone
    (Depo-Provera)
  Levonorgestrel (Norplant)

The progestin-only oral contraceptive, Norplant, and Depo-Provera are recommended over combined (estrogen and progestin) oral contraceptives. Combined oral contraceptives have been noted to decrease milk output significantly and cause foul-smelling stools and gastrointestinal distress in some infants. Progestin-only preparations have not been associated with decreased milk supply if begun after lactation is fully established.

73. Define weaning.

The discontinuation of breast-feeding; the infant or child receives all his or her nourishment through other sources.[5]

74. How is weaning accomplished?

In **infant-initiated weaning**, the mother follows the infant's cues. The mother neither offers nor denies the infant the breast. Gradually the infant decreases his or her breast-feeding pattern.

Mother-initiated weaning occurs when the mother ends breast-feeding despite the infant's desire to continue to breast-feed.

Gradual weaning also is initiated by the mother. The mother is advised to remove one breast-feeding session approximately every 3 days. This time allows adjustment to the change in feeding pattern and allows the mother's breast milk supply time to adjust. To substitute for the feeding, the mother can offer the child a snack, drink, or diversion. Over a period of weeks or months, the mother can decrease the frequency of breast-feeding slowly until the child eventually stops completely. By allowing time for a gradual weaning, the mother is able better to adjust physically and emotionally to the discontinuation of breast-feeding.[5]

CONTROVERSIES

75. Can a mother with hepatitis C virus (HCV) breast-feed?

The reported rates of vertical transmission via delivery vary, but the risk of HCV infection via breast milk is low. The recommendation for breast-feeding in the presence of HCV is controversial. If the titer levels are low, the benefits of providing breast milk to the infant born to an HCV-positive mother may outweigh the risks. The health care provider should discuss the risks of HCV versus the benefits of breast feeding.

76. Discuss the current recommendations for a HIV-positive mother and breast-feeding.

HIV is transmitted through blood and body secretions. Transmission of HIV may occur prenatally, during birth, and during the postpartum period. There has been some documentation in the literature of transmission through breast milk. Based on the limited information available, the current recommendation is to advise women known to be HIV-1 positive not to breast-feed. In communities where the primary causes of death are malnutrition and infectious diseases, however, breast-feeding is encouraged and supported. The benefits of breast-feeding must outweigh the risks. In these communities, the risk of HIV infection through breast milk transmission is likely to be lower than the risk of death from malnutrition or an infectious disease. Any woman who is HIV positive should consult a health care provider regarding the choices for feeding her infant.

BIBLIOGRAPHY

1. American Academy of Pediatrics Work Group on Breastfeeding: Breastfeeding and the use of human milk. Pediatrics 100:1035–1039, 1997.
2. American College of Obstetricians and Gynecologists: Breastfeeding: Maternal and Infant Aspects. ACOG Educational Bulletin No. 258. Washington, DC, ACOG, 2000.
3. Association of Women's Health, Obstetric and Neonatal Nurses: Standards and Guidelines for Professional Nursing Practice in the Care of Women and Newborns, 5th ed. Washington, DC, AWHONN, 1998.
4. Hale T: Medications and Mother's Milk, 9th ed. Amarillo, TX, Pharmasoft Publishing, 2000.
5. Lauwers J, Shinskie D: Counseling the Nursing Mother: A Lactation Consultant's Guide, 3rd ed. Boston, Jones & Bartlett, 2000.
6. Lawrence R: Breastfeeding: A Guide for the Medical Professional, 5th ed. St. Louis, Mosby, 1999.
7. Mohrbacher N, Stock J: LaLeche League International: The Breastfeeding Answer Book. Schaumburg, IL, LaLeche League International, 1997.
8. Newman J: Breastfeeding problems associated with the early introduction of bottles and pacifiers. J Hum Lactation 6:59–63, 1990.
9. Newman J: How breast milk protects newborns. Sci Am 273:76–79, 1995.
10. Riordan J, Auerbach K: Breastfeeding and Human Lactation, 2nd ed. Sudbury, MA, Jones and Bartlett, 1998.
11. Shrago L, Bocar D: The infant's contribution to breastfeeding. J Obstet Gynecol Neonat Nurs 19:209–215, 1990.
12. Slusser W, Powers N: Breastfeeding update 1: Immunology, nutrition, and advocacy. Pediatr Rev 18:111–119, 1997.
13. Tully M: Recommendations for handling of mother's own milk. J Hum Lactation 16:149–151, 2000.
14. WHO/UNICEF Statement: Ten Steps to Successful Breastfeeding: Protecting, Promoting, and Supporting Breastfeeding: The Special Role of Maternity Services. Geneva, World Health Organization, 1989.

7. RESPIRATORY SYSTEM

Lauren R. Sorce, RN, MSN, CCRN, CPNP,
Andrea Kline, RN, MS, CCRN, PCCNP, *and Joyce Weishaar*, RN, MSN, CCNS

1. List common signs of respiratory distress in children.
Nasal flaring
Tracheal tugging
Retractions (suprasternal, intercostal, subcostal)
Head bobbing

2. What is the first step in evaluating a patient with respiratory distress?
Determine whether the causative area is in the upper airway or lower airway.

3. How can the nurse differentiate between upper and lower airway obstruction on physical examination?

	UPPER AIRWAY OBSTRUCTION	LOWER AIRWAY OBSTRUCTION
Respiratory rate	Slow	Slow
Duration of inspiratory phase	Increased	Increased or decreased
Duration of expiratory phase	Increased or decreased	Increased
Stridor	Present	Absent
Wheezing and gas trapping	Absent	Present

4. What clinical situation should be suspected in children with sudden onset of respiratory distress associated with coughing, gagging, stridor, or wheezing?
Foreign body aspiration.

5. List objects that may be aspirated by children.

Coin (most common object)	Hot dogs
Balloons	Grapes
Toys	Candies
Peanuts	Other small objects

6. What test is done to diagnose a foreign body aspiration?
A **radiographic examination**. Approximately 90% of foreign bodies are radiopaque. Radiographic examination can determine the location, type, and number of objects in the ingestion. Contrast administration or fluoroscopy may be necessary to identify some objects, such as plastic toys or parts.

7. Where is the appropriate place to deliver back blows to an infant with a foreign body aspiration?
Using the heel of the hand, deliver back blows between the shoulder blades.

8. What is bronchiolitis?
An acute inflammatory process resulting in obstruction of small airways.

9. List causative agents of bronchiolitis.
Respiratory syncytial virus (RSV) (most common)
Adenovirus
Influenza

Rhinovirus
Parainfluenza virus type 3
Mycoplasma pneumoniae (older children)

10. When does bronchiolitis occur?

Bronchiolitis is more common in the winter months when viruses are more commonly problematic.

11. Why is RSV a problematic virus?

1. RSV causes inflammation and infiltration of the bronchiolar epithelium, which leads to submucosal edema and necrosis, resulting in mucus plugging of small airways with cellular debris and atelectasis.

2. RSV is an extremely hardy virus and easily transmitted. It lives on hands for 25 minutes, latex gloves for 1.5 hours, and countertops for 6 hours.

3. Because of its easy transmission, nearly all children by the age of 3 have had RSV.

4. RSV is particularly virulent in children with other diseases, such as congenital heart disease, immunodeficiency, metabolic diseases, neurologic diseases, cystic fibrosis, chronic lung disease, and other chronic illnesses.

12. Name other risk factors for RSV.

1. Premature infants and infants < 6 weeks old are at high risk for RSV infection.

2. Boys are at higher risk for hospitalization than girls because they seem to have more severe symptoms.

3. Children from a low socioeconomic status are at increased risk for hospitalization, likely as a result of overcrowding and frequent exposures.

4. Children who require hospitalization for other reasons are at risk for RSV resulting from nosocomial infection.

13. Can RSV bronchiolitis be fatal?

Yes. Annual mortality statistics are as follows:
• Approximately 1% of previously healthy children
• 3.5% of children with cardiac or pulmonary disease
• 20–67% of immunocompromised children

14. List the signs and symptoms of RSV bronchiolitis.

Rhinitis	Malaise	Retractions
Increased work of breathing with retractions	Irritability	Prolonged expiratory phase
	Pharyngitis	Wheezing
Fever	Anorexia	Rales
Tachypnea	Cough	Apnea
Hypoxemia	Dyspnea	

In small infants, **apnea** may be the first sign of illness.

15. How is RSV bronchiolitis diagnosed?

Diagnosis is by history and physical examination, pulse oximetry, RSV testing, and chest radiograph.

The **history** includes information about the signs and symptoms. The child likely has been exposed to other ill people, attends day care or school, or has been exposed to other crowded conditions.

Pulse oximetry shows desaturated blood as a result of atelectasis and small airway plugging (if the airways are closed or plugged, gas exchange cannot occur across the alveolar membrane).

RSV testing can be done, and although commonly positive, some children may be infected with other viruses or bacteria.

Chest radiograph shows hyperinflation (too much air in the lungs), streaky quality to the lungs, and atelectasis.

16. Discuss the treatment of bronchiolitis.

Treatment is supportive because most cases are of viral origin. Dehydration should be treated with **oral rehydration therapy** or **intravenous therapy** if the child is dehydrated as a result of difficulty eating or bottle feeding with respiratory symptoms or excessive insensible losses as a result of tachypnea, fever, and increased work of breathing. Other therapies include **oxygen delivery** and **bronchodilators** as needed. The use of **steroids** in the treatment of bronchiolitis is controversial because of opposing results in research studies. If the causative agent is RSV, treatment of the hospitalized child with **ribavirin** is controversial because of conflicting research outcomes.

17. Discuss medications to reduce the risk of occurrence of RSV bronchiolitis.

There currently is no vaccination or immunization for bronchiolitis. There is a medication, however, which when given monthly can reduce the risk of contracting RSV. **Palivizumab** is a humanized monoclonal antibody that has been proved to decrease hospitalization resulting from RSV by 55%. Palivizumab should be given to children who meet the recommended criteria. **RSV immunoglobulin** is an immunoglobulin derived from human immunoglobulins that also has decreased hospitalization by 41%. RSV immunoglobulin also has recommended criteria for administration. Palivizumab has become the preferred choice because it is administered by the intramuscular route monthly, whereas RSV immunoglobulin must be administered intravenously each month.

18. What is pneumonia?

An infection in the lungs caused most frequently by bacteria or virus. It results in an inflammatory process that progresses to alveolar consolidation, reduced lung compliance, and decreased vital capacity and total lung capacity. In children, pneumonia is the most common life-threatening illness.

19. List the signs and symptoms of pneumonia.

Fever	Dyspnea
Cough	Tachypnea
Rhinorrhea	Tachycardia
Congestion	Cyanosis
Poor appetite	Crackles and diminished aeration
Increased work of breathing	over the area of consolidation

20. How is pneumonia diagnosed?

- Pneumonia is most commonly diagnosed by **chest radiograph**. Different types of pneumonia can look different on the radiograph.
- **History and physical examination** also are helpful in diagnosing pneumonia.
- **Cultures** of the sputum may be sent to identify a causative organism.
- A **complete blood count** with an elevation of white blood cells is suggestive of infection.
- If the causative organism originated in the blood (bacteremia), a **blood culture** may be helpful with identification of the organism.
- For children with severe illness, other diagnostic tests, such as **lung biopsy** or **bronchoalveolar lavage**, may be done to identify the causative agent.

21. Discuss the treatment for pneumonia.

Treatment depends heavily on the causative agent. If the agent is bacterial, **antibiotics** are prescribed. If the agent is viral, treatment is **supportive**. Other types of causative agents, such as fungi, may be treated with appropriate medications. If needed, **oxygen therapy** is initiated. **Rehydration therapy** is given if the child is dehydrated from poor intake of fluids, fever, and increased work of breathing, all of which increase insensible losses of fluid from the body.

22. How can you tell the difference between laryngotracheobronchitis/croup and epiglottitis?

	LARYNGOTRACHEOBRONCHITIS/CROUP	EPIGLOTTITIS
Cause	Viral	Bacterial
Age	2 mo–3 y	2–6 y
Pathology	Glottic, subglottic, tracheal, bronchial edema	Edema of epiglottis and surrounding area
Onset	Gradual	Acute
Signs and symptoms	Sore throat, hoarseness, barky cough, stridor, low-grade temperature, retractions	High temperature, sore throat, dysphagia, dysphonia, drooling, stridor, distress, sniffing position
Diagnosis	History and physical examination, radiograph	History and physical examination, radiograph
Lateral neck radiographs	Steeple sign	Thumb print
Treatment modalities	Oxygen, mist, racemic epinephrine nebulizer; steroids; heliox; airway management	Antibiotics, airway management may be emergent; blood cultures after airway secured

23. Discuss special concerns regarding the child with epiglottitis.

1. Care should be taken to keep the child **comfortable** by providing an oxygen delivery system that is least noxious to child and decreasing the performance of noxious procedures (e.g., removing the scared child from his or her parent, intravenous access). The child is at risk for **complete airway closure** should he or she do anything (e.g., cry, fight) to compromise the already at-risk airway. Never perform an oral exam on a child with suspected epiglottitis.

2. If the child has **severe respiratory distress** and requires **endotracheal intubation**, this should be done in the operating room by clinicians *most* skilled in airway management. If endotracheal intubation is not successful, an emergent **tracheotomy** must be performed to provide an airway for the child.

24. How prevalent is asthma in the pediatric population?

It is the most common chronic disease in children and the most prevalent reason for a visit to the emergency department. Of all children, 5–10% are affected with some symptoms of asthma. It occurs more frequently in boys than girls until the teen years, when occurrence becomes equal. Most children with asthma experience their first symptoms before the age of 5 years.

25. Name the causes of airway obstruction in asthma.

Airway edema
Acute bronchoconstriction
Production of mucous plugs

26. List some asthma triggers.

• Exposure to dust mites, roaches, cigarette smoke, paint fumes, air pollution, or solvents
• Allergies to animal dander, outdoor seasonal molds, and airborne pollens
• Viral infections or gastroesophageal reflux
• Weather changes, especially humidity and temperature

27. What does a child look like when having an asthma exacerbation?

Airway obstruction occurs during expiration—there is distal airway trapping or hyperinflation. An asthma exacerbation is characterized by increased work of breathing, as is evidenced by nasal flaring and intercostal retractions. On auscultation, there is decreased air movement. Although expiratory wheeze is a common symptom, it is not an exclusive symptom of asthma. There is a prolonged expiratory phase, with high-pitched, musical inspiratory sounds. Tachypnea and cough are present. The child is restless and anxious. As the exacerbation progresses, color changes from dusky to cyanotic; agitation increases; and the child has difficulty speaking, needing to pause frequently to breathe.

28. Describe a good way to measure the severity of asthma exacerbations.

Peak expiratory flow rate (PEFR) measures the child's ability to push air forcefully out of fully inflated lungs and is the maximal rate of expiration. A baseline measurement is obtained and is documented as the personal best measurement. Children younger than 5 years of age have difficulty with this manner of measurement. Measurements during an exacerbation can be grouped according to zones, and plan of care and treatment is designed according to the zone of measurement:

    Green zone   80–100% of personal best
    Yellow zone   50–80% of personal best
    Red zone   < 50% of personal best; this is a **medical alert**, and the child should be **hospitalized**.

29. What are the goals of treatment of asthma?

To reverse the symptoms, reduce the incidence of exacerbations, and maintain as close to normal pulmonary functioning as possible. These goals are accomplished by avoiding or controlling exposure to triggers, assessing lung function and severity of exacerbations (PEFR is done easily at home), using the right medication or combination of medications for maintenance therapy and treatment of exacerbations, and comprehensive patient and family education.

30. What types of drugs are available for asthma?

MEDICATION	USES

Anti-inflammatory agents
  Cromolyn (Intal)
  Nedocromil (Tilade)
	Used to inhibit early-phase and late-phase allergen bronchospasm
	Not bronchodilators

Corticosteroids
  Oral prednisone
  Intravenous steroids
  Inhaled beclomethasone
    (Beclovent)
	Control seasonal allergies and exercise-induced asthma only if other therapies fail
	Preferably used on an alternate-day schedule to reduce side effects
	Short courses used for exacerbations

β_2-Adrenergic agonists
  Albuterol
  Terbutaline
	Relax airway smooth muscle and enhance mucociliary clearance
	Agents of choice for acute exacerbations or daily therapy
	Increased use of as-needed doses indicates need to increase therapy
	Long-acting β_2-adrenergic agents (e.g., salmeterol [Serevent]) not used for exacerbations

Anticholinergic agents Ipratropium (Atrovent)	Potent bronchodilators Less effective than β_2-adrenergic agents but can be used in conjunction with them
Bronchodilators with mild anti-inflammatory effects Theophylline	Not commonly used Significant adverse side effects, such as tachycardia, gastrointestinal symptoms, and seizures Used when inhaled steroids and β_2-adrenergic agents fail to control symptoms Need to monitor levels to maintain within therapeutic limits

31. Give a classification of asthma with treatment according to severity.

CATEGORY	CHARACTERISTICS	TREATMENT
Mild	Symptoms are present $\leq 2 \times$/wk PEFR $\geq 80\%$ personal best	No daily medications. use of short-acting β_2-agonists no more than 2–3 ×/wk
Mild persistent	Exacerbations > 2/wk but < 1 d PEFR $\geq 80\%$ personal best	Daily long-term antiinflammatory agent such as cromolyn Use of β_2-agonists for exacerbations. If use increases to daily, go to next category.
Moderate persistent	Exacerbations > 2/wk that may last for ≥ 24 h PEFR 60–80% personal best	Daily antiinflammatory agents. May add long-acting bronchodilator. For exacerbations, β_2-agonist for relief not to exceed 3–4 ×/d.
Severe	Continuous symptoms Frequent exacerbations PEFR $\leq 60\%$ personal best	Daily: inhaled high-dose steroids *plus* sustained-release theophylline or β_2 agonist (or both) For exacerbations, continued as- needed use of β_2 agonists

32. When is hospitalization for asthma necessary?

When symptoms are refractory to treatment, the PEFR is < 70% of personal best, or the patient is high risk (i.e., previous history of hospitalization for asthma or intubation).

33. What can the nurse do to prepare the patient and family for discharge?

Education is the key—the family and patient need to be aware of asthma triggers and to make changes in the home environment to limit exacerbations. General information about asthma and specific information about the child's status should be given. The use and proper administration of medications is vital. Education should focus on what to do if additional use of β_2-agonists increases, how to treat exacerbations, and monitoring peak flow with return demonstration. The goal is to limit exacerbations and the need for hospitalization.

34. What is cystic fibrosis?

The most common lethal, hereditary disorder in the United States. It is caused by the defective activation of a cyclic adenosine monophosphate–dependent ion channel. A simultaneous increased reabsorption of sodium occurs, with intraluminal fluid dehydration.

35. Describe the clinical manifestations of cystic fibrosis.

Clinical manifestations occur in the lungs, pancreas, intestinal tract, and liver. The **respiratory symptoms** predominate with thick mucus production, chronic respiratory infections, and inflammation. Poor-to-absent exocrine function of the **pancreas** leads to malabsorption and resultant poor somatic growth. **Liver failure** and **diabetes** also may occur.

36. How is cystic fibrosis treated?

- Respiratory symptoms often are managed with bronchodilators, mucolytics, and postural drainage.
- Lung-heart, single or double organ, transplantation may be considered in children with end-stage disease. Transplantation currently is being performed with moderate success.
- Because of malabsorption, these patients generally receive vitamin supplementation, including vitamins A, D, E, and K.

37. What is the most common diagnostic test used to evaluate a patient for cystic fibrosis?

The **sweat chloride test**. This test is simple but has a high rate of false-positive and false-negative results when performed by an inexperienced laboratory. Concentrations of sodium and chloride in the sweat are low (< 40 mEq/L) in individuals without cystic fibrosis and generally are high (> 60 mEq/L) in patients with cystic fibrosis.

38. What is the most common modality used in managing respiratory disease?

Oxygen therapy.

39. Name four ways to deliver oxygen.

1. Oxygen mask (facemask)
2. Face tent
3. Oxygen hood
4. Nasal cannula

40. Describe the simple facemask.

This is a low-flow device that delivers 35–50% oxygen with a flow rate of 6–10 L/min. Typically the patient's inspiratory flow rate exceeds that of the delivery system, and subsequent oxygen dilution occurs with entrainment of gas flow through side ports on the mask.

41. Describe the partial rebreather facemask.

This is a facemask with a reservoir bag and gas inflow system. There is no one-way valve mechanism. The mask can deliver reliably an inspired oxygen concentration of 50–60%.

42. Describe the nonrebreather facemask.

This facemask incorporates a mask, reservoir bag, and gas inflow system. Exhaled gases are eliminated, and each breath consists of fresh gas. This mask features a valve incorporated into the exhalation port to prevent entrainment of room air on inspiration and a valve placed between the reservoir bag and the mask to prevent exhaled gas from entering the bag. This facemask can deliver the highest amount of oxygen of all of the facemasks. It can deliver 100% oxygen, provided that the gas flow in the reservoir system is adequate to maintain bag distention throughout the entire respiratory cycle.

43. Describe the face tent.

This is a soft plastic bucket that often is tolerated better in children than the facemask. Reliable delivery of oxygen concentration greater than 40% generally cannot be provided. A benefit of the face tent is accessibility to the patient's mouth for procedures such as suctioning without interruption in oxygen delivery.

44. Describe the oxygen hood.

This is a plastic shell that surrounds the patient's head. It is well tolerated by infants and allows access to the patient's chest and trunk. It also permits the control of inspired flow of oxygen, gas, temperature, and humidity. Because of oxygen hood size limitations, the oxygen hood may used in children younger than 1 year old.

45. Describe the nasal cannula.

This consists of two prongs that are inserted in the anterior aspect of the nares. Oxygen is provided into the nasal pharynx, operating at flow rates of 0.1–6 L/min. The inspired oxygen concentration is influenced by nasal resistance, inspiratory flow rate, and tidal volumes. Exogenous humidification is not provided with a nasal cannula. The nasal cannula generally can deliver 25–50% oxygen, but it is difficult to monitor the exact concentration being administered.

46. What percent of oxygen does room air contain, and what gas comprises the rest of room air?

Room air is 21% oxygen and 79% nitrogen.

47. What helpful information does a pulse oximeter provide?

The pulse oximetry monitor is an important noninvasive technique used to evaluate a child's oxygen saturation. It does not measure adequacy of ventilation (carbon dioxide elimination), but it may provide an early indication of respiratory deterioration and development of hypoxemia. The pulse oximeter requires pulsatile blood flow and does not provide useful data in a child with poor perfusion or shock.

48. Discuss care of the patient after receiving a new tracheostomy.

The new tracheostomy tube must be secure for the first 4–7 days after surgery to enable a tract to form between the trachea and the skin. Stay sutures (sutured to each side of the new tracheal incision and taped to the chest) are frequently in place after surgery and are used to open the trachea in case of decannulation, but it may be difficult to reinsert the tube. Tracheostomy ties go around the neck and are secured to the tracheostomy tube. They generally are made of twill tape or Velcro (a beaded metal tie also is available). Tracheostomy ties need to be fastened so that the caregiver can insert at least the tip of one finger between the child's neck and the tie. Especially with children, care must be taken with Velcro ties because the child could unfasten them easily and decannulate. With the presence of the tracheostomy, filtering and humidification functions of the nose and throat are bypassed so that humidified oxygen and air must be administered to prevent dryness of the respiratory mucosa. Although secretions may be blood-tinged at first, large amounts of bloody secretions are uncommon.

49. Discuss suctioning a tracheostomy.

The goal of suctioning is to clear and maintain a patent airway with the least amount of trauma from the procedure. A patient is suctioned as needed (whenever secretions pool and cause difficulty breathing), not at preplanned intervals. In general, the largest catheter that advances in the tube allows thick tenacious secretions to be evacuated. Sterile technique is used in the hospital setting, and clean technique is reserved for the home. Previously the technique used to suction was to insert the catheter until resistance was met, withdraw slightly, then apply suction. This technique has been found to cause inflammation and denuded epithelium. The premeasured technique now is used, which causes less damage by measuring the depth of catheter insertion to be no more that 0.5 cm beyond the end of the tube. Length of time to apply suction should be no more than 15 seconds. It helps if you hold your own breath at the start of suctioning so that you have an idea how long the child is deprived of air. If you have to breathe, the child also needs air. Allow 30–60 seconds between passes to allow oxygenation to return to normal. If the patient's oxygen saturations fall, ventilate with oxygen between passes to maintain saturations.

50. How often is the tracheostomy changed?

The physician usually does the first tracheostomy change 5–7 days after the surgery. After that, the frequency varies according to institution or physician preference from weekly (most common) to twice weekly. Advantages of more frequent tracheostomy changes are keeping the caregiver familiar with the procedure so that he or she is comfortable with it, decreased airway infections, and relief of a partially obstructed tube (dried secretions can adhere to the side of the tube). Disadvantages to frequent changing are patient discomfort and possible stretching of the stoma with cuffed tracheostomy tubes. It is recommended that a smaller tube be available in case of problems with insertion; if a child has little reserve, a smaller tube can be inserted to expedite ventilation. Check ventilation after tube insertion because the tube could be inserted into the soft tissues surrounding the trachea.

51. What kind of problems may a child with a tracheostomy experience?

• Accidental decannulation may occur at any time. Another tracheostomy tube and ties need to be available at all times, along with a manual resuscitation bag in case it is needed.

• The tracheostomy can plug with secretions as evidenced by increased work of breathing (use of accessory muscles, nasal flaring), color change, anxiety, and restlessness. Immediate suctioning should take place. If ventilation does not improve, even with manual ventilation, change the tracheostomy tube. If all else fails, the child can be ventilated with bag and mask while occluding the stoma.

• Tracheal wall erosion, tracheoinnominate artery fistula, stomal breakdown, tracheomalacia, and recurrent tracheitis and bronchitis can occur. The longer the tracheostomy is in place, the more likely it is that complications will occur.

52. What does the family need to know before taking the child with a tracheostomy home?

1. Two caregivers should be identified for intensive education so that one always will be available.

2. The caregivers need to be taught about any equipment used and to be able to set it up and take it apart.

3. Care of the tracheotomy, such as stoma care, suctioning, and tracheostomy change, should be modeled using a doll or mannequin. After the caregivers have practiced their techniques, they should perform the technique on the child.

4. Respiratory assessment and signs and symptoms of illness should be taught.

5. **Cardiopulmonary resuscitation (CPR)** should be taught, using resuscitation bag-to-tracheostomy and mouth-to-mouth resuscitation, should the provider be unable to reinsert the decannulated tracheostomy.

6. Encourage the caregivers to take over the care of the child during hospitalization so that they become familiar with a routine.

7. A **go-bag** should always be with the child; it contains portable suction, suction catheters, extra tracheostomy tube and ties, manual resuscitation bag, and emergency phone numbers.

8. Mock emergency situations should be practiced so that caregivers will know how to respond.

9. Before discharge, the caregivers may stay overnight, rooming in, and assume full responsibility for the child's care with the nurse as a resource and observer, not participant.

BIBLIOGRAPHY

1. American Thoracic Society: Care of the child with a chronic tracheostomy. Am J Respir Crit Care Med 16:297–308, 2000.
2. Ball J, Bindler R (eds): Pediatric Nursing: Caring for Children, 2nd ed. Stamford, CT, Appleton & Lange, 1999.
3. Behrman R, Kliegman R (eds): Nelson Essentials of Pediatrics, 3rd ed. Philadelphia, W.B. Saunders, 1998.
4. Breese Hall C: Respiratory syncytial virus: A continuing culprit and conundrum. J Pediatr 135(suppl):S2–7, 1999.
5. Burns C, Brady M, Dunn A, Stack N (eds): Pediatric Primary Care: A Handbook for Nurse Practitioners, 2nd ed. Philadelphia, W.B. Saunders, 2000.
6. Chameides L, Hazinski MF (eds): Pediatric Advanced Life Support. Dallas, TX, American Heart Association, 1997.
7. Curley MAQ, Moloney-Harmon P (eds): Critical Care Nursing of Infants and Children, 2nd ed. St. Louis, Mosby, 2001.
8. Darville T, Yamauchi T: Respiratory syncytial virus. Pediatr Rev 19:55–61, 1998.
9. Davis B, Lagrone C: Nursing education: Streamlining discharge planning for the child with a new tracheostomy. J Pediatr Nurs 12:191–192, 1997.
10. Englund JA: Prevention strategies for respiratory syncytial virus: Passive and active immunization. J Pediatr 135(suppl):S38–44, 1999.
11. Harkin H: Tracheostomy management. Nursing Times 95:56–58, 1998.
12. Rodriguez WJ: Management strategies for respiratory syncytial virus infection in infants. J Pediatr 135(suppl):S45–50, 1999.
13. Rogers MC, Nichols D (eds): Textbook of Pediatric Intensive Care, 3rd ed. Baltimore, Williams & Wilkins, 1996.
14. Rudolph AM (ed): Rudolph's Pediatrics, 20th ed. Stamford, CT, Appleton & Lange, 1996.
15. Slota MC: Core Curriculum for Pediatric Critical Care Nursing. Philadelphia, W.B. Saunders, 1998.
16. Wong D (ed): Whaley and Wong's Essentials of Pediatric Nursing, 5th ed. St. Louis, Mosby, 1997.

8. CARDIOVASCULAR SYSTEM

Deborah Bibeau, RN, MSN

1. What changes occur in the heart and circulation at birth?

1. The **lungs** take over the role of oxygenating the blood.

2. The **patent ductus arteriosus (PDA)** closes functionally in the first week as a result of increased arterial oxygenation.

3. The **foramen ovale** closes because left atrial pressure exceeds right atrial pressure, closing the flap valve of the foramen.

4. **Pulmonary vascular resistance** drops rapidly in the first hour of life and gradually over the next 4–6 weeks.

2. Describe the normal course of blood flow through the heart.

Unoxygenated blood enters the heart through the superior and inferior venae cavae into the right atrium. The blood then enters the right ventricle through the tricuspid valve and is pumped to the lungs through the pulmonary valve and pulmonary arteries. Oxygenated blood returns to the left atrium from the lungs by the pulmonary veins. The blood is pumped into the left ventricle through the mitral valve, then out to the body through the aortic valve and the aorta.

3. List some indications of cardiac dysfunction that can be obtained from the patient history.

Decreased exercise tolerance
Varying degrees of cyanosis
Dizziness or syncope
Respiratory difficulties
Repeated respiratory infections
Delays in physical growth and development
Chest or limb pain
Palpitations
Edema

4. List signs of decreased exercise tolerance in children.

• Excessive fatigue or shortness of breath with normal activities
• Unable to keep up with peers during normal activities
• Need to stop and rest frequently
• Tendency to choose more quiet activities

5. What is a sign of exercise intolerance in infants?

Infants may become excessively fatigued, may become breathless, or may sweat excessively during feedings.

6. List signs and symptoms of respiratory difficulties.

Congested cough   Retractions
Rapid respirations   Nasal flaring
Grunting respirations

7. Name the measurements of cardiac function.

Heart rate   Stroke volume
Blood pressure   Pulmonary vascular resistance
Cardiac output   Systemic vascular resistance

8. Give age-related normal heart rate and blood pressure values.

AGE	HEART RATE (BEATS/MIN)	SYSTOLIC PRESSURE (mmHg)	DIASTOLIC PRESSURE (mmHg)
Newborn	91–182	64–78	41–52
1–6 mo	103–186	95–110	58–71
6–11 mo	109–170	95–110	58–71
1–2 y	95–165	95–110	58–71
3–6 y	65–140	101–115	57–68
7–11 y	62–130	104–124	55–82
12–15 y	60–130	112–138	62–83

9. What is the most accurate way to count the heart rate?

The **apical pulse**, which is counted using a stethoscope. It should be taken for 1 full minute. When the auscultated apical rate is greater than the palpated radial pulse, the difference is called a **pulse deficit**.

10. What are the important things to remember when measuring blood pressures?

1. Make sure the blood pressure cuff is the right size. Use the largest size that fits comfortably on the extremity being used.

2. The pressures in the legs normally should be slightly higher than the pressures in the arms.

3. Four extremity blood pressures should be checked in any child with suspected heart disease. Pressures that are lower in the legs than the arms may indicate a **coarctation of the aorta**.

11. List signs of cardiac disease that can be assessed just by looking at the child.

Decreased activity level   Chest deformities
Lethargy   Clubbing
Squatting posture   Edema
Cyanosis   Increased respiratory effort
Bulging neck veins   Retractions

12. What is cyanosis?

A bluish discoloration of the skin and mucous membranes resulting from decreased oxygen concentration in the arterial blood. The level of hemoglobin influences the ability to detect cyanosis. Cyanosis is more apparent in patients with **polycythemia** than in patients with anemia.

13. How does cyanosis differ from acrocyanosis?

Acrocyanosis is a normal finding in newborns. It usually is seen as a blueness of the hands and feet and is related to vasoconstriction from the cold.

14. List some points to consider when assessing pulses.

- **Femoral pulses** are important to check. Decreased strength of femoral pulses may indicate a coarctation.
- **Weak pulses** are associated with a partial occlusion of the artery or decreased cardiac output.
- **Water-hammer (Corrigan's) pulse** is forceful and jerky and associated with a wide pulse pressure.
- **Pulsus alternans** is an alteration of weak and strong pulses without changes in the cycle length.

- **Paradoxical pulse** is an exaggeration of the normal variation of pulse intensity. The pulse gets weaker with inspiration and stronger with expiration.
- In **sinus arrhythmia**, the pulse rate increases with inspiration and decreases with expiration.

15. Explain what causes the different heart sounds.

The heart sounds are produced by the opening and closing of the heart valves and the action of blood against the walls of the heart and vessels.

- S_1 is caused by the closure of the mitral and tricuspid valves.
- S_2 is caused by the closure of the aortic and pulmonic valves. It normally splits with inspiration and closes with expiration.
- S_3 sometimes is heard in early diastole (just after S_2) and is caused by blood flowing from the atria into the ventricles and is due to diastolic overload of the ventricles or decreased ventricular compliance.
- S_3 and S_4 are **gallops**.
- S_4 is heard late in diastole (just before S_1) and is due to decreased compliance of the ventricles.
- **Ejection clicks** occur in systole and indicate abnormal semilunar valves.
- **Opening snaps** occur early in diastole and indicate abnormal atrioventricular valves.
- **Friction rubs** are scraping or squeaking sounds that occur when the pericardial sac becomes inflamed and rubs against the heart.
- **Murmurs** are caused by the turbulence of blood flow as it passes through the heart; they can be normal or abnormal.

16. How do you describe heart murmurs?

Grade or intensity describes how loud the murmur is.

- Grade I is faint and requires careful listening.
- Grade II is quiet but readily heard.
- Grade III is moderately loud with no associated thrill.
- Grade IV is loud with an associated thrill.
- Grade V is loud with an associated thrill and can be heard with the stethoscope partially off the chest wall.
- Grade VI is loud with an associated thrill and can be heard with the stethoscope off the chest wall.

Timing describes where in the cardiac cycle the murmur is heard.

- Systolic murmurs are heard between S_1 and S_2.
- Diastolic murmurs are heard between S_2 and S_1.
- Continuous murmurs are heard throughout systole and diastole.

Location is the anatomic location where the murmur is heard the loudest.

Frequency or quality of the murmur is how the murmur sounds.

• High-pitched	• Vibratory
• Medium-pitched	• Crescendo
• Low-pitched	• Decrescendo
• Blowing	• Crescendo-decrescendo

17. Name characteristics of a murmur that would suggest a pathologic murmur.

• Diastolic murmur	• Loud murmur
• Associated thrill	• Holosystolic murmur

18. What causes congestive heart failure (CHF)?

CHF is failure of the heart to pump adequately and is caused by increased volume, obstruction to outflow, ineffective myocardial function, excessive demands for cardiac output, or arrhythmias.

19. List the signs and symptoms of CHF.

Tachycardia	Fatigue	Cyanosis	Neck vein distention
Tachypnea	Hypotonia	Hacking cough	Nausea
Hepatomegaly	Flaccidity	Hypotension	Anorexia
Cardiomegaly	Dyspnea	Grunting	Ascites
Gallop rhythm	Retractions	Nasal flaring	Irritability
Oliguria	Edema	Sweating	Lethargy
Diaphoresis	Pallor	Rales	Fever
Slow growth	Mottling		

20. Describe the types of medications that may be used to treat CHF.

Diuretics (furosemide, thiazides) can be used to decrease fluid retention. The type of diuretic used usually is determined by the severity of the CHF.

Inotropic agents (digoxin, dobutamine) are used to increase the contractility of the heart.

Vasodilators can be used to improve left ventricular function by decreasing preload and afterload. Angiotensin-converting enzyme (ACE) inhibitors are vasodilators used in long-term treatment of CHF. ACE inhibitors block the conversion of angiotensin I to angiotensin II. Angiotensin II acts as a vasoconstrictor and raises the blood pressure by increasing venous return and sodium and water retention.

Phosphodiesterase inhibitors (amrinone, milrinone) have inotropic and vasodilator effects. They improve cardiac function by increasing contractility.

21. List other treatments for CHF.
- Oxygen therapy
- Rest
- Weight reduction
- Fluid and electrolyte management
- Elimination of the precipitating factors
- Mechanical ventilation (in patients with severe CHF to minimize the work of breathing)

22. Define preload.

Preload is the amount of stretch that occurs in the heart muscle as a result of the load placed on the muscle before contraction. It is related to the amount of blood that fills the heart at the end of diastole.

23. Define afterload.

Afterload is the resistance against which the heart must pump and is related to the blood pressure and vascular resistance.

24. Describe the normal conduction system of the heart.

The conduction impulse originates in the **sinoatrial node**, then spreads through both atria. The impulse is delayed by the **atrioventricular node** to allow the atria to contract and fill the ventricles before the ventricles contract. The atrioventricular node sends the impulse via the bundle of His, the right and left bundle branches, and the Purkinje fibers to the ventricles.

25. How is the electrocardiogram (ECG) in the infant and child different from that in the adult?

In newborns, the right ventricle has more muscle mass than the left ventricle. This appears on the ECG as right-axis deviation and tall or large R waves in leads aVR, V_1, and V_2. There are deep S waves in leads I, V_5, and V_6. The T wave in the right precordium (V_{4R}, V_1) should be inverted from about 2 days to 8–10 years of age. The P wave, P-R interval, and QRS durations all are prolonged during childhood. The ECG progresses to showing left ventricular dominance by adulthood.

26. Show normal ECG values by age.

ECG Normals by Age

AGE	P-R (SEC)	QRS (SEC)	R IN V$_1$ (MM)	S IN V$_1$ (MM)	R IN V$_6$ (MM)	S IN V$_6$ (MM)
Newborn	0.08–0.15	0.03–0.08	3–26	0–23	0–16	0–10
1–6 mo	0.08–0.15	0.03–0.08	3–20	0–15	5–22	0–10
6–11 mo	0.07–0.16	0.03–0.08	2–20	0.5–20	6–23	0–7
1–2 y	0.08–0.16	0.03–0.08	2–18	0.5–21	6–24	0–7
3–6 y	0.09–0.17	0.04–0.08	1–18	0.5–24	4–26	0–4
7–11 y	0.09–0.17	0.04–0.09	0–14	0.5–25	4–25	0–4
12–15 y	0.09–0.2	0.04–0.1	0–14	0.5–21	4–25	0–4

27. What are the most common pediatric arrhythmias?

The most common significant pediatric arrhythmias are **supraventricular tachycardia** (SVT) and **paroxysmal atrial tachycardia**. Sinus arrhythmia is so common that it is really considered a normal variant in children. Premature atrial and ventricular contractions also are common.

28. How do you treat SVT in children?

A 12-lead ECG should be obtained in any stable child with SVT before any attempts at treatment. Initially, attempts to stop SVT with vagal maneuvers may be made. These maneuvers may include ice to the face, rectal temperatures, gagging, carotid massage, Valsalva maneuvers, or headstands. If these maneuvers do not work, the next step is the administration of adenosine. If at any time the patient's condition deteriorates because of the tachycardia, **cardioversion** is used to restore the normal rhythm.

29. What is radiofrequency catheter ablation?

A special type of catheterization procedure that is used to eliminate an abnormal pathway that causes SVT. The first part of the procedure is diagnostic, the electrophysiology study. During electrophysiology study, the exact location and characteristics of the abnormal pathway are identified. During the second part of the procedure, the abnormal pathway is eliminated by burning the cells with radiofrequency energy. This burn creates scar tissue that no longer can conduct electrical impulses.

30. Describe management of SVT in children.

The first-line **antiarrhythmic** used in children with SVT is usually a β-blocker. Digoxin commonly was used in the past, but its efficacy has been questioned. Otherwise, management depends on the characteristics of the tachycardia, the age of the patient, the severity of symptoms, and any concurrent conditions.

31. List things to keep in mind when administering adenosine.

- Adenosine should be given with a physician present.
- The normal dosing is 50–250 µg/kg.
- Adenosine must be given rapidly because of its short half-life of only a few seconds.
- Adenosine blocks conduction through the atrioventricular node.
- Older children may feel heaviness in their chest or get short of breath and should be warned.
- Adenosine may cause bronchospasm and should be used with caution in asthmatics.

32. Are heart rates in the 40s abnormal for children?

In younger children, yes; however, healthy athletic adolescents often have normal heart rates in the 40s. Any rate at which a child is symptomatic for **bradycardia** with low cardiac output or low blood pressure is considered too low and may require therapy. Often, bradycardia is secondary to hypoxemia, apnea, or increased vagal tone.

33. What is the youngest age at which a pacemaker can be implanted?

Current pacemakers have been made smaller with advances in technology. Pacemakers now can be implanted in premature infants. Infants and younger children who require pacemakers usually have **epicardial pacemaker systems** implanted.

34. Describe the different types of pacemaker systems.

Dual-chamber pacemakers sense or pace in the atrium and the ventricle, whereas **single-chamber pacemakers** sense or pace only in one or the other.

Endocardial systems involve threading the leads into the heart through the great vessels, whereas **epicardial systems** use leads attached to the outside of the heart muscle.

35. State the risk of development of congenital heart disease (CHD) in the general population.

CHD occurs in about 1% of the general population. This risk increases to about 3% if there is a first-degree relative with CHD and may be 10% in children of parents with CHD.

36. List factors that contribute to an increased risk of developing CHD.

- Maternal infections, such as rubella, cytomegalovirus infection, coxsackie infection, and herpes infection
- Diabetes
- Poor nutrition
- Alcohol use
- Drugs, such as anticonvulsants, lithium, progesterone, estrogen, and warfarin
- Genetic disorders
- Family history of cardiac disease

37. List genetic disorders that usually have associated CHD.

DiGeorge syndrome	Turner's syndrome
Down syndrome	Klinefelter's syndrome
Trisomy 18	Cri du chat syndrome
Trisomy 13	

Other genetic causes of CHD are being recognized every year.

38. List other syndromes that have associated CHD.

Specific gene defects have not yet been characterized for the following syndromes, but may be recognized in the future.

- CHARGE association (*c*oloboma of the eye, *h*eart anomaly, choanal *a*tresia, *r*etardation, *g*enital anomalies, *e*ar anomalies)
- Congenital diaphragmatic hernia
- Cornelia de Lange's syndrome
- Fetal alcohol syndrome
- Fetal hydantoin syndrome
- Fetal trimethadione syndrome
- Fetal warfarin syndrome
- Infant of a diabetic mother
- Pierre Robin syndrome
- VATER/VACTERL syndrome (*v*ertebral, *a*nal, *c*ardiac, *t*racheal, *e*sophageal, *r*enal, and *l*imb)

39. Name five cyanotic CHD lesions.

1. Tetralogy of Fallot
2. Tricuspid atresia
3. Transposition of the great arteries
4. Total anomalous pulmonary venous return
5. Pulmonary atresia

40. Name acyanotic CHD lesions.

PDA	Atrioventricular septal defect
Coarctation of the aorta	Pulmonic valve stenosis
Ventricular septal defect (VSD)	Aortic stenosis
Atrial septal defect	

41. What interventional catheterization techniques can repair or improve certain defects?
- **Coils** can be used to occlude extra vessels such as PDAs.
- **Balloons** are used to open up stenotic valves or to dilate narrow vessels.
- **Stents** can be used to open up vessels and maintain their patency.
- **Intra-arterial occlusion devices** or **septal occluders** can be inserted to close atrial septal defects.
- **Surgical blades** can be used to create connections, such as in atrial septal defects.
- **Radiofrequency energy catheters** can be used to eliminate abnormal electrical pathways and can be used to open atretic valves.

42. What lesions are associated with tetralogy of Fallot?

VSD	Overriding of the aorta over the VSD
Pulmonary stenosis	Enlarged right ventricle

43. How is tetralogy of Fallot treated?
Tetralogy of Fallot (TOF) is treated surgically. Children usually undergo repair around 6 months to 1 year of age. Surgical repair involves closing the VSD with a patch, removing any muscle obstructing the flow of blood, and opening the pulmonary valve if narrowed.

44. Define hypoplastic left heart syndrome.
Hypoplsatic left heart syndrome (HLHS) results when the side of the heart that pumps the blood to the body is underdeveloped. This includes an underdeveloped aorta and left ventricle and underdeveloped or absent aortic and mitral valves.

45. What are the treatment options for hypoplastic left heart syndrome?
Three-stage Norwood procedure and heart transplant.

46. Define subacute bacterial endocarditis (SBE).
SBE is an infection of the endocardial tissue and usually involves the heart valves. Endocarditis often causes leakage of valves, and emboli can cause multiple organ failure.

47. Name the leading cause of death in SBE.
CHF.

48. How can the risk of SBE be reduced?
By having at-risk patients take an antibiotic before dental, gastrointestinal, and genitourinary procedures. The antibiotic dose recommended is a larger dose than that given for other infections and is given one time, 1 hour before the procedure.

49. Which cardiac lesions require SBE precautions?
All CHDs except secundum atrial septal defects. Abnormal or prosthetic valves also are at risk.

50. List dosing ranges for some of the commonly used cardiac medications.

MEDICATION	DOSAGE
Atenolol	1–2 mg/kg/day
Captopril	0.1–1.4 mg/kg q 8 hr

Table continued on following page

MEDICATION	DOSAGE
Digoxin	8–10 µg/kg/day
Furosemide	1–2 mg/kg/dose 1–3 times/day
Potassium chloride	1–2 mEq/kg/day

51. List signs of digoxin toxicity.

Bradycardia	Vomiting	Dizziness
Arrhythmias	Headache	Confusion
Anorexia	Drowsiness	Visual disturbances
Nausea	Insomnia	

52. List common side effects of ACE inhibitors.

Hypotension	Neutropenia	Elevated liver enzymes
Hyperkalemia	Gastrointestinal irritation	Chronic dry cough
Rash	Loss of taste	Renal dysfunction

53. What are the important points to teach families about compounded medications?

• Patients and families need to be shown how to draw up the dose of medication.
• Patients and families need to follow the directions for storage on the bottle.
• These preparations need to be mixed thoroughly before drawing up the dose because the medication may settle in the suspension and affect how much medication is actually being given with each dose.
• Patients and families should know the dosage in milligrams and milliliters because different pharmacies may make up the medication in different concentrations.

CONTROVERSY

54. Should four-extremity blood pressures be part of a well-child visit?

Performing four-extremity blood pressure measurements may seem impractical for the general pediatric practice. A study by Ing et al. concluded, however, that a blood pressure differential is the most consistent finding in children with **coarctation of the aorta**. Their study showed that early detection and repair of coarctation of the aorta greatly reduced hypertensive problems in adulthood. They recommended "that all children should be screened for coarctation of the aorta by measuring blood pressure in the upper and lower extremities during at least one routine examination during infancy and certainly before 3 years of age; any child with elevated blood pressure should be specifically evaluated for coarctation of the aorta, because this is the most common cause of remediable hypertension in the pediatric population."

BIBLIOGRAPHY

1. Allen HD, Gutgesell HP, Clark EB, Driscoll DJ (eds): Moss and Adams' Heart Disease in Infants, Children, and Adolescents, 6th ed. Philadelphia, Lippincott Williams & Wilkins, 2001.
2. Clark BJ, Ramaciotti C, Chang A: Cardiology. In Polin RA, Ditmar MF (eds): Pediatric Secrets, 2nd ed. Philadelphia, Hanley & Belfus, 1997, pp 53–78.
3. Engel J: Pocket Guide to Pediatric Assessment, 2nd ed. St. Louis, Mosby, 1993, pp 148–160.
4. Guzzetta CE, Dossey BM (eds): Cardiovascular Nursing: Holistic Practice. St. Louis, Mosby, 1992.
5. Ing FF, Starc TJ, Griffiths SP, Gersony WM: Early diagnosis of coarctation of the aorta in children: A continuing dilemma. Pediatrics 98:378–382, 1996.
6. Olsen GP, Driscoll D: Circulation: Implications of abnormalities in structure and pressure. In Mott SR, Frazekas NF, James SR (eds): Nursing Care of Children and Families: A Holistic Approach. Menlo Park, CA, Addison-Wesley, 1985, pp 1155–1218.
7. Park MK: Pediatric Cardiology for Practitioners, 3rd ed. St. Louis, Mosby, 1996.
8. Stillwell SB, Randall EM: Pocket Guide to Cardiovascular Care, 2nd ed. St. Louis, Mosby, 1994.

9. NEUROLOGIC SYSTEM

Delia R. Nickolaus, RN, MSN

1. At what point in gestation does the neural tube close?
By the 28th day of gestation. This is before most women know they are pregnant.

2. Why is folic acid supplementation important for all women of child-bearing age?
Folic acid supplementation of 400 µg/day can prevent neural tube defects by 70%.

3. List the most common congenital anomalies of the central nervous system.
1. Hydrocephalus (1–2 per 1000 births)
2. Spina bifida, a neural tube defect (1 per 1000 births)
3. Craniosynostosis (1 per 2000 births)

4. State some facts about the presence of cerebrospinal fluid (CSF) in the ventricular system and its importance.
- CSF is produced at a rate of approximately 20 mL/hr in a normal child.
- Total volume in the infant's ventricular system is approximately 50 mL and gradually increases with age to 150 mL in the adult.
- CSF volume is maintained by a balance in the secretion and absorption of the CSF.
- CSF is secreted primarily by the choroid plexus.
- CSF is absorbed primarily by the arachnoid villa.
- CSF provides protection for the brain and spinal cord and delivers nutrients and removes wastes.

5. When is hydrocephalus usually detected?
Some cases are detected **in utero** when the enlarged ventricles are noted on ultrasound. Most cases are detected through **routine screening** by the family pediatrician when the child's head circumference jumps above the normal growth curve. All children younger than 2 years old should have their head circumference monitored by the primary care physician.

6. Describe communicating (or nonobstructive) hydrocephalus.
Communicating hydrocephalus is caused by an impairment of the secretion/absorption balance of CSF leading to excessive volume within the ventricular system. It is seen most commonly in children with spina bifida, intraventricular hemorrhages, meningitis, and brain trauma.

7. Describe noncommunicating (or obstructive) hydrocephalus.
Noncommunicating hydrocephalus is caused by a mass or some other physical blockage of the CSF flow leading to an increase in the fluid volume within a particular area of the ventricular system. It usually is seen with tumors, trauma, some cases of spina bifida, and structural anomalies such as aqueductal stenosis.

8. List treatment options for hydrocephalus.
- **Ventriculoperitoneal shunt**—a thin tube and valve under the skin from the ventricles to the peritoneal space.
- **Ventriculoatrial shunt**—a thin tube and valve under the skin from the ventricles to the right atrium of the heart.
- **Ventriculostomy** of the third ventricle—a small hole surgically placed in the base of the third ventricle of the brain.

9. What is spina bifida (myelomeningocele)?

Failure of the neural tube to close completely during the first 28 days of gestation leads to a fluid-filled sac containing neural elements that protrudes from the opening in the vertebral column resulting in varied degrees of neural damage. It is seen most frequently in the lumbosacral area.

10. How is spina bifida diagnosed?

Maternal serum alpha-fetoprotein blood test or ultrasound by at least the 20th week of gestation.

11. How does spina bifida affect the child?

Neurologic. Hydrocephalus requiring CSF diversion is present in 80% of children. Variable levels of developmental delay occur. Degree of mobility is based on the level of the spinal lesion. Chiari II malformation is seen in approximately 99% of children.

Urologic. Dysfunctions occur requiring varying degrees of intervention ranging from medications, to clean intermittent catheterizations, to surgical interventions.

Orthopedic. Multiple and varied conditions occur, including hip dislocation, scoliosis, kyphosis, short stature, and weakened bones.

Varying degrees of **endocrine** problems occur.

Latex sensitivity develops secondary to exposure to latex products through numerous surgical procedures.

12. List treatment options for parents who are told their fetus has spina bifida.
- **Termination** of the pregnancy
- **Early delivery** at 34–36 weeks' gestational age with closure of the myelomeningocele within 48 hours to prevent infection and further neurologic damage
- **Intrauterine closure** of the myelomeningocele; this treatment option is still experimental

13. What is craniosynostosis?

Premature closure of one or more cranial sutures.

14. What causes craniosynostosis?

The cause of **primary craniosynostosis** is unknown, although 10–20% of cases are associated with genetic syndromes. **Secondary craniosynostosis** is caused by failure of the brain to grow and expand. Neurologic outcomes are based on the underlying cause of the craniosynostosis.

15. When do the fontanels normally close?
- The posterior fontanel closes by 8 weeks of age.
- The anterior fontanel closes by 18 months of age.
- By 12 years of age, the cranial sutures are closed such that they cannot be separated by an increase in intracranial pressure.

16. Name the key components of the neurologic examination.
- Extensive **history** from family and patient, as appropriate.
- Observe **behavior**: interaction with parents, play patterns.
- **Physical examination** in a nonthreatening atmosphere.
- Observe for outward **physical characteristics** (e.g., shape of the head, low-set ears).
- Cranial nerve assessment
- Motor examination
- Sensory assessment

17. How do you assess the 12 cranial nerves?

MNEMONIC	NERVE NUMBER	CRANIAL NERVE	FUNCTION AND ASSESSMENT
On	I	Olfactory	Smell: Test sense of smell with something familiar to the child; test each nostril individually
Old	II	Optic	Vision: Check child's visual acuity with a Snellen chart. Check peripheral vision. Use ophthalmoscope to check ocular fundus
Olympus	III	Oculomotor	Extraocular eye movement and elevation of eyeball; pupil constriction and dilation: Check pupil size and reactivity to light. Check position of eyelid when eye is open. Have the child follow an object through the six cardinal positions of gaze
Towering	IV	Trochlear	Upward and downward movement of the eyeball: Have the child look downward and upward with the eyes
Top	V	Trigeminal	Sensation of face and chewing: Have patient clench teeth; test for facial sensation by using a light touch on each cheek, forehead, and jaw
A	VI	Abducens	Lateral eye movement: Assess ability of child to look sideways
Finn	VII	Facial	Facial expression and taste: Observe ability to smile showing teeth, puff out cheeks. Assess sense of taste for sweet, sour, and bitter on the anterior portion of the tongue
And	VIII	Auditory/acoustic	Hearing: Localize to voice; attend to finger rub
German	IX	Glossopharyngeal	Taste, pharyngeal sensation, and swallowing: Assess the child's ability to taste sweet, sour, and bitter on the posterior one third of the tongue. Test gag reflex by touching wall of pharynx. Watch uvula and soft palate while client says "aah"
Viewed	X	Vagus	Larynx and pharynx sensation: Assess for hoarseness and ability to swallow. Check gag reflex
Some	XI	Spinal accessory	Head and shoulder movement: Have the child turn head to the side against resistance. Assess strength of shoulder shrug
Hops	XII	Hypoglossal	Tongue movement: Assess if tongue is midline and the ability to move tongue from side to side. Assess for tongue strength, by having child push against tongue blade with tongue.

NOTE. When assessing the cranial nerves, accommodations should be made for the child's age and developmental ability to follow directions.

18. What is a traumatic brain injury (TBI)?
Injury to the brain that may be localized to one area of the brain or diffuse, depending on the mechanisms of injury.

19. Which age group is at increased risk for TBI?
Children < 5 years old.

20. List mechanisms of TBI most commonly seen in children.

Motor vehicle crashes	Gunshot wounds
Falls	Child abuse

21. How is TBI exhibited?
The sequelae of the injury depend on the area of the brain where the injury occurred and the extent of the damage.

REGION OF THE BRAIN	BEHAVIORS RELATED TO INJURY
Frontal	Emotional lability
Parietal	Aphasia, deficits in writing, math, self-care skills
Temporal	Auditory and visual disturbances, impaired long-term memory, altered personality
Occipital	Visual-perceptual deficits
Cerebellar	Balance, coordination, nystagmus
Brainstem	Basic consciousness, breathing

22. What education is needed by the child and family after any head injury?
1. Recovery from any head injury may take a few weeks to ≥ 12 months depending on the severity of the injury.
2. Depending on the degree of injury, there may be long-term effects on motor function, memory, cognition, communication skills, and psychosocial adaptation.
3. Neuropsychologic evaluation may be helpful in some cases for early detection of problems.
4. Individual state laws determine the extent of the programs available to a child after a TBI.

23. In which area of the spine do pediatric spinal cord injuries occur?

Infancy to 8 years of age	75% of injuries occur in the cervical spine, most frequently the upper cervical spine.
8–14 years of age	60% of injuries occur in the cervical spine, 20% occur in the thoracic spine, and 20% occur in the thoracolumbar spine.
> 14 years of age	Injuries are similar to injuries that occur in adults with an even split between cervical and thoracolumbar spine injuries.

24. What is the most common cause of pediatric spinal cord injuries?
Forty-five percent of all injuries result from **motor vehicle crashes**.

25. What is the most common pediatric brain tumor?
Astrocytomas account for 50% of all pediatric brain tumors.

26. Name the other tumors that account for 50% of pediatric brain tumors.

Medulloblastoma	Craniopharyngioma
Ependymoma	Brainstem glioma

27. List descriptive characteristics of astrocytoma.

1. Astrocytomas may be benign or malignant depending on the cell pathology.

2. Astrocytomas in the cerebellum, hypothalamus, optic chiasm, and optic nerve are most often benign.

3. Astrocytomas of the brainstem are most often malignant.

4. Astrocytomas of the cerebral hemispheres have an even occurrence of malignant versus benign pathology.

28. Describe the usual primary treatment for pediatric brain tumors.

Surgical resection of the tumor is the primary treatment. This may be done as one surgery or in several stages based on the tumor size and location and tumor type. Advances with **magnetic resonance imaging–guided surgery** prevent injury to normal brain tissue that surrounds the tumor. **Radiation therapy** and **chemotherapy** are used in conjunction or instead of the surgery based on the tumor's pathology.

29. What is posterior fossa syndrome?

A relatively rare syndrome seen at least 24 hours postoperatively when the surgical tumor resection involves the posterior fossa area of the brain. The cause is not fully understood.

30. List signs and symptoms of posterior fossa syndrome.
- Mutism or some degree of speech disturbances
- Dysphagia
- Motor weakness
- Emotional lability
- Cranial nerve palsies

31. What are some particular concerns regarding posterior fossa syndrome?

Recovery may take days to months depending on the severity. The patient and family need extensive support in coping with this syndrome, especially the speech disturbances, communication, and emotional lability issues.

32. State some facts that differentiate seizures and epilepsy.

1. Seizures have the highest incidence of all neurologic dysfunctions.

2. Seizures are abnormal electrical discharges within the brain caused by some underlying disease process.

3. Epilepsy is a chronic seizure disorder with recurrent seizures of unknown origin.

33. Name the most common first-line antiseizure medications and their dosages.

Phenobarbital: 15–20 mg/kg as a loading dose; maintenance dose, 1–6 mg/kg/day in one to two divided doses based on age of the child.

Phenytoin (Dilantin): 15–20 mg/kg loading dose; maintenance dose, 5–10 mg/kg/day in two to three divided doses based on the age of the child.

Diazepam (Valium): 0.2–0.5 mg/kg for children > 2 years old for acute seizure activity; dosage based on age of the child.

Lorazepam (Ativan): 0.05–0.1 mg/kg for acute seizure activity; dosage based on age of the child.

34. State some facts about headache occurrence among school-age children.
- Tension-type headache is the most common.
- Twenty percent of all children in the United States aged 5–17 suffer from chronic headaches.
- Seventy-five percent of children with chronic headaches suffer from tension-type headaches.

35. What is the difference between occasional headaches and chronic headaches?
- Occasional headaches occur once or twice a month.
- Chronic headaches occur two or more times per week.

• Children who develop chronic headaches should be evaluated by the primary care practitioner for treatment.

36. How are tension headaches differentiated from migraine headaches?
• **Tension headaches** frequently are caused by stress, inadequate rest, environmental triggers, or food triggers.
• **Migraine headaches** usually have a family history.
• Children who experience car or motion sickness are more likely to develop migraine headaches, especially if there is a family history of migraines.
• Migraine headaches occur in 25% of children who suffer from chronic headaches.

37. List methods of treatment for pediatric headaches.
• Over-the-counter medications such as acetaminophen, ibuprofen, and naproxen sodium can be used for relief of symptoms.
• Prescription medications, such as amitriptyline, may be used as a preventive intervention.
• Alternative and adjunct methods, such as ice packs, sleep or rest in a dim room, warm bath or shower, and massage, may be particularly helpful with a tension-type headache.
• Manage stress through relaxation techniques and biofeedback.
• Teach the family and patient to recognize and avoid headache triggers.

38. List signs that, in association with a headache, require immediate evaluation by a medical team member.

Loss of balance or coordination	Weakness
Increased time spent sleeping	Stiff neck accompanied by a fever
Seizure activity	Nausea and vomiting
Loss of consciousness	Visual changes
Personality change	

39. What is attention deficit hyperactivity disorder (ADHD)?
The inability to attend to a task, accompanied by increased motor activity and impulsivity.

40. State some general facts about ADHD.
1. Oppositional and aggressive behaviors often are seen together with ADHD.
2. Children with ADHD also may have some learning disabilities.
3. The cause of ADHD is currently unknown.
4. Prevalence is approximately 3–5% in school-age children.
5. ADHD is seen four times more frequently in boys than in girls.

41. When is ADHD diagnosed?
• Initial concerns usually arise when the child starts school.
• The child is disruptive and unresponsive to directions in a school-like setting.
• The child does not seem to learn from negative consequences and continues with the disruptive behavior.

42. How is ADHD treated?
Psychosocial: Implement a daily routine; a few simple, clear rules; and firm limits that are enforced.
Pharmacologic: Methylphenidate (Ritalin) and dextroamphetamine (Adderall) are used most commonly.
Drug-free periods during weekends, holidays, and summer vacations are important to reassess the continued need for pharmacologic treatment.

43. Discuss cerebral palsy.

Cerebral palsy is the most common permanent physical disability of childhood. It occurs approximately 1.5–3 times per 1000 live births and has multifactorial causes. The most predominant risk factor is premature delivery. *Cerebral palsy* is a nonspecific term applied to disorders characterized by early onset of impaired movement and posture with accompanying developmental impairment.

44. List the clinical manifestations of cerebral palsy.
- Altered motor movement that may involve increased tone, decreased tone, tremors, and ataxia
- Variable degrees of developmental disabilities, including possible hearing, visual, speech, cognitive, and behavioral involvement
- Possible seizure activity

BIBLIOGRAPHY

1. Behrman RE, Kliegman RM, Jenson HB: Nelson's Textbook of Pediatrics, 16th ed. Philadelphia, W.B. Saunders, 2000.
2. Children's headaches: An informative guide for young sufferers, their parents, and school health professionals. Available at http://www.headaches.org/educationalmodules/childrensheadaches/ chhome.html.
3. Cheek WR, Marlin AE, McLone DG, et al (eds): Pediatric Neurosurgery: Surgery of the Developing Nervous System. Philadelphia, W.B. Saunders, 1998.
4. Cunningham FG, MacDonald PC, Leveno KJ, et al: Williams Obstetrics, 19th ed. Norwalk, CT, Appleton & Lange, 1993.
5. Engel J: Pocket Guide to Pediatric Physical Assessment, 2nd ed. St. Louis, Mosby, 1993.
6. Hockenberry-Eaton M (cd): Essentials of Pediatric Oncology Nursing: A Core Curriculum. Glenview, IL, Association of Pediatric Nurses, 1998.
7. Merestein GB, Kaplan DW, Rosenberg AA: Handbook of Pediatrics, 18th ed. Stamford, CT, Appleton & Lange, 1997.
8. Pilliteri A: Child Health Nursing: Care of the Child and Family. Philadelphia, Lippincott Williams & Wilkins, 1999.
9. Siberry GK, Iannone R (eds): The Harriet Lane Handbook: A Manual for Pediatric House Officers, 15th ed. St. Louis, Mosby, 2000.
10. Taketomo CK, Hodding JH, Kraus DM: Pediatric Dosage Handbook, 7th ed. Hudson, OH, Lexi-Comp, 2000.
11. Wong DL, Hockenberry-Eaton M, Wilson D, et al: Wong's Essentials of Pediatric Nursing, 6th ed. St. Louis, Mosby, 2001.

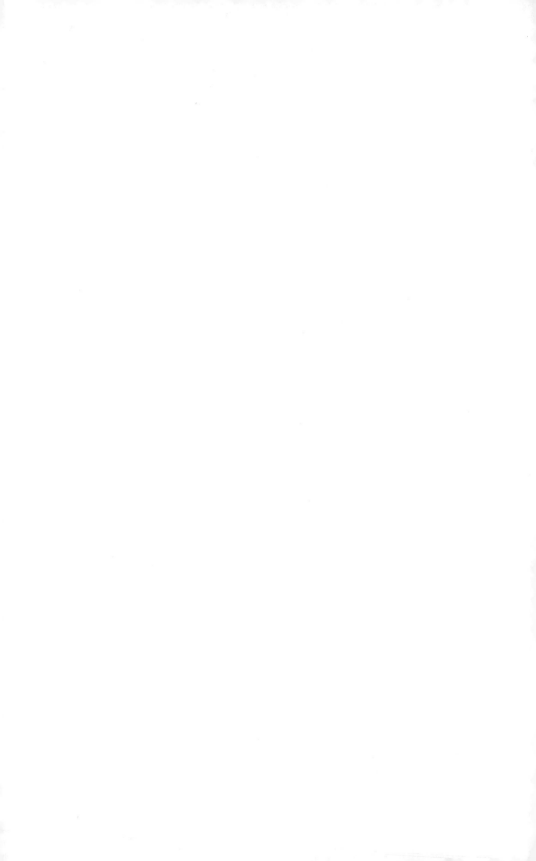

10. GASTROINTESTINAL SYSTEM

Barbara Hoyer Schaffner, PhD, RN, CPNP

1. Discuss possible causes of acute abdominal pain in children.

Most pain is from a self-limiting disease. Clues to determine the cause of the abdominal pain may come from the history. Reports of pain that interrupts the child's usual activity, pain that worsens over time, and pain that manifests in an ill-appearing child who is lying still and refusing to move onto or off the examination table require intense evaluation for an acute abdominal process.

2. Summarize the evaluation of acute abdominal pain.

QUESTIONS	POSSIBLE CAUSE
Is there evidence of trauma?	Child abuse Accidental injury
Is there a history of fever?	Urinary tract infection Streptococcal pharyngitis Gastroenteritis Viral syndrome Mononucleosis Pneumonia
Middle to left-sided abdominal pain?	Constipation Torsion of the ovary or testicle
Middle to right-sided abdominal pain?	Appendicitis Ovarian torsion Testicular torsion Mittelschmerz
Abdominal pain present in other family members?	Food poisoning Viral syndrome Gastroenteritis
Blood in the stool?	Inflammatory bowel disease Hemolytic-uremic syndrome Gastroenteritis
Blood in the urine?	Stones Renal trauma Urinary tract infection
Evidence of obstruction?	Malrotation Intussusception
Sexually active?	Sexually transmitted disease Pelvic inflammatory disease Ectopic pregnancy

3. When does abdominal pain become recurrent or chronic?

Recurrent abdominal pain is defined as three episodes of abdominal pain in 3 months in children between the ages of 4 and 16 years.

4. What is the incidence of recurrent abdominal pain?
- Recurrent abdominal pain affects about 14% of school-age children.
- It is more common in girls between 9 and 10 years old and boys 10–11 years old.

5. How do you differentiate organic from inorganic abdominal pain?
Indicators of **inorganic** abdominal pain:
- Pain in periumbilical or epigastric areas that does not radiate
- Rarely awakens from sleep
- May have problems falling asleep
- May keep eyes closed during physical examination of abdomen

Indicators of **organic** abdominal pain:
- Pain located away from the midline
- Pain is nocturnal, especially if it awakens the child in the middle of the night
- Persistent emesis
- Pain related to meals
- Diarrhea or blood in the stool
- Extraintestinal symptoms, such as fever, rash, and joint aches
- Involuntary weight loss or lack of linear growth
- Abnormal urinalysis or culture
- School attendance regular despite recurrent pain
- Eyes open during the examination

6. Discuss the difference between gastroesophageal reflux (GER) and gastro-esophageal reflux disease (GERD).

GER is a physiologic phenomenon causing occasional spitting up in infants owing to the immaturity of the muscle tone in the gastrointestinal tract of infants. The problem resolves spontaneously without intervention in most cases by the time the infant is sitting and standing upright.

GERD is a chronic condition that causes damage to the mucosa of the esophagus of the infant or child.

7. What are the characteristics of GER?

GER usually is seen in infants (newborns to 12–18 months old). The infant has a continuous history of regurgitation with every feed. There are no risk factors that increase the likelihood of an infant having GER; it can occur in any newborn. The infant with GER has symptoms isolated to GER without the complications of pain or respiratory disorders. The infant continues to gain weight and grows along a normal growth curve for length and birth weight. When GER is suspected in isolation, there is no need for further diagnostic evaluation.

8. How is GER in infants treated?

Treatment consists of feeding the infant with frequent thickened feedings.

9. How do the signs and symptoms of GERD differ in infants and children?

Infants experience the characteristic regurgitation seen with GER. Infants may suffer from irritability, painful swallowing with a resultant refusal to eat, and heartburn from the esophagitis. Some infants and children experience a slowing or stopping of growth, exhibiting failure to thrive. For some infants, GERD causes respiratory disorders, such as stridor, lower respiratory disease, and apnea. Posturing, with neck contortions, has been observed in some infants. GERD resolves in most cases by the age of 2 years.

In older children, GERD takes on a pattern similar to that in adults, with GERD becoming persistent and chronic. Esophagitis is a major problem with pharmacologic interventions frequently needed. Older children often have a respiratory component to their symptoms, including frequent respiratory disorders, wheezing, and a diagnosis of asthma.

10. What other disease entities might be confused with GERD?

SYSTEM	DISORDER	
Gastrointestinal	Regurgitation, vomiting	Esophagitis
	Dysphagia	Intestinal obstruction
	Peptic ulcer disease	Pyloric stenosis
Respiratory	Central apnea	Inflammatory disorders
	Obstructive disorders	Infectious disorders
Cardiac	Pain of cardiac origin	
Musculoskeletal	Costochondritis	
Neurologic	Seizure disorders	Nonspecific infant irritability
	Sandifer's syndrome	

11. Discuss treatment of GERD.

Treatment initially consists of conservative recommendations regarding **positioning** and **feeding**. In severe cases, **pharmacologic therapy** and **surgery** may be recommended.

Positioning of infants in the prone position while awake and side lying or on their back when sleeping is advised. Elevation of the head of the bed often is suggested, but the research on an elevated positioning of infants with GERD has failed to find a significant improvement in symptoms.

Feeding interventions are the cornerstone of GERD treatment. It is recommended that 1 tablespoon of dry cereal be added to every 1–2 oz of formula. The formula should be thick enough to necessitate the enlargement of the nipple to allow adequate flow of formula. For older children, avoidance of fatty foods, acidic juices, carbonated drinks, coffee, and alcohol is advised. Older children should be encouraged to avoid eating before bedtime, to maintain a normal weight for age and height, to avoid tight clothing, and to avoid contact with second-hand smoke.

If necessary, **pharmacologic therapy** may include over-the-counter antacids. Adult GERD medications, including histamine H_2 receptor antagonists, proton-pump inhibitors, and prokinetic agents, have not been approved by the Food and Drug Administration for pediatric use. Referral to a gastroenterologist is indicated when conservative treatment with positioning and feeding interventions is ineffective.

12. Discuss the approach to a child who is vomiting.

Vomiting usually is preceded by nausea in the verbal child. Many diseases of diverse origins can cause vomiting, and the clinical findings obtained through history and physical examination usually provide clues. Sustained vomiting can cause signs and symptoms, such as lethargy, tachycardia, poor skin turgor, and decreased urinary output, that are seen with dehydration.

13. List causes of vomiting.

SIGN	POSSIBLE CAUSE
If spitting up without fever	Regurgitation
	Reflux
	Inappropriate feeding (overfeeding)
	Nervous vomiting
If spitting up with fever	Viral gastroenteritis
	Otitis media
	Other infections
If spitting up with fever and diarrhea	Viral gastroenteritis
	Food poisoning

Continued on following page

SIGN	POSSIBLE CAUSE
If projective vomiting with signs of intestinal obstruction	Pyloric stenosis Intussusception Hernia Adhesion Peptic ulcer Appendicitis
If projective vomiting with abnormal neurologic examination	Central nervous system injury Shaken baby syndrome
If projective vomiting with poor growth	Diabetes Renal disease Metabolic disease
If projective vomiting with poor growth and on medications	Theophylline Erythromycin Digitalis
If vomiting and sexually active	Pregnancy
If vomiting, no fever, no weight loss, no diarrhea, not sexually active	Psychogenic Migraine

14. What is colic?

A syndrome of crying in infants who in all other ways appear healthy and are growing and developing normally. The infant who has colic usually is less than 3 months old and has episodes of excessive inconsolable crying for no apparent reason. The crying can begin at 1 month of age. Most infants cry at the same time day, most commonly in the evening, and have been described as turning red, firming their abdominal wall, and drawing up their legs.

15. When is colic a correct diagnosis?

Colic is the correct diagnosis only *after* the infant has been examined thoroughly, current growth rate has been confirmed, and all other causes of the crying have been eliminated.

16. What is intussusception?

The most common cause of intestinal obstruction in young children, age 3 months to 5 years; it is seen most commonly in boys 3–12 months old.

17. Describe the signs and symptoms of intussusception.

The classic presentation is a healthy thriving infant that suddenly develops an attack of acute, colicky abdominal pain. The infant typically screams and draws the legs up toward the chest. The pain is intermittent, and the infant may act normal in between painful episodes. The infant also may vomit during times of pain. The classic **currant jelly stool** appears later on in the disease process and is associated with a tender and distended abdomen.

18. How is intussusception treated?

Treatment consists of a **nonsurgical hydrostatic reduction** through barium enema; if this is unsuccessful, surgery is indicated.

19. Define Hirschsprung's disease.

A congenital anomaly that results in an aganglionic megacolon causing a mechanical obstruction of the intestine from inadequate motility of the aganglionic section. In the newborn period, failure to pass a meconium stool in the first 24–48 hours of life is indicative of Hirschsprung's disease.

20. Describe the stool pattern of the infant and child with Hirschsprung's disease.

Infants show patterns of constipation associated with abdominal distention. **Children** show chronic constipation with the occasional passing of a ribbonlike foul-smelling stool. Poor growth is present in all children from birth.

21. Discuss possible causes of rectal bleeding.

Rectal bleeding is a fairly common manifestation of gastrointestinal disease because the rectum is the final pathway of hemorrhage from any site along the gastrointestinal tract. The color, location, and amount of blood are important in determining the cause. Bright red blood or bloody streaking of the stool is usually from lesions low in the gastrointestinal tract, such as **fissures** or **polyps**. **Meckel's diverticulum** may produce red bleeding, whereas **currant jelly stools** are a classic sign of **intussusception**. Bloody stools with **mucus** may be due to infection, food or milk allergies, ischemia, Hirschsprung's disease, or colitis. **Melena** usually is associated with upper gastrointestinal bleeding.

22. List causes of rectal bleeding by age.

AGE	CAUSES OF RECTAL BLEEDING	
Newborn–3 mo	Swallowed maternal blood	Upper gastrointestinal tract bleeding
	Nasopharyngeal trauma	Hemorrhagic disease of the newborn
	Anal fissures	Anatomic abnormalities
3 mo–3 yr	Infection	Esophagitis
	Anal fissure	Lymphoid hyperplasia
	Milk or soy allergy	Peptic ulcer or gastritis
	Colonic polyp	Structural abnormalities
	Intussusception	Hemolytic-uremic syndrome
	Antibiotic-related colitis	Vascular abnormalities
	Meckel's diverticulum	
3–18 yr	Infection	Peptic ulcer or gastritis
	Polyps	Varices
	Anal fissures	Lymphoid hyperplasia
	Inflammatory bowel disease	Vascular lesions

23. What do normal stools look like in infancy?

The first bowel movement an infant has is thick and dark green or black in color. A breast-fed infant has yellowish loose, seedy stools. A formula-fed infant has yellowish to tan stools that are similar in texture to peanut butter. As long as the infant is feeding well and wetting the diaper well, there is no need for concern if the infant does not have a bowel movement every day. After the newborn period, the color of the stool depends on the type of formula, how often and how much the infant eats, and if breast-fed what the mother is eating. The number of bowel movements decreases in infants between 1 and 12 months old. The color of the stool changes based on what the infant eats and is not of concern unless the color is black, red, or white.

24. Define constipation in infants.

Constipation is having hard, dry stools that are formed, come out in pellets, or look and feel like marbles. Pushing, grunting, straining, and crying with bowel movements are common in infants, even when the stools are soft.

25. How should infant constipation be treated?

- If an infant is constipated, giving 1–2 oz of prune or pear juice twice a day adds fiber to the infant's diet.

• If the infant is older than 4 months, adding infant food high in fiber content, such as prunes, peaches, pears, plums, peas, or spinach, twice a day may help.
• Use of infant glycerin suppositories is appropriate if dietary intervention is unsuccessful.

26. What about constipation in children?

Constipation occurs in 5–10% of children. Most constipation in children is a **functional disorder**, and few children require referrals to gastroenterologists.

27. How should childhood constipation be treated?

Therapy includes altering the child's diet, bowel training, laxatives, and disimpaction.

Dietary management should include a high-fiber diet to add bulk and increase bowel peristalsis. A generous amount of fluid should be encouraged, but milk, apple juice, and tea should be limited to two 8-oz glasses each day.

Bowel training emphasizes bowel retraining and includes having the child sit on the toilet twice a day for extended periods (10–20 minutes) usually in the morning and evening after meals (at the same time every day). It is helpful if the child can place his or her feet flat on the floor.

The use of **laxatives** can include mineral oil or milk of magnesia. Other over-the-counter products, such as the **natural laxatives**, senna, cascara, and casanthranol, have been found to be gentle and safe for long-term use in children.

Enemas can be included in the treatment plan to relieve fecal impactions within the rectum.

28. Define diarrhea.

An increase in frequency or decrease in consistency of the stool.

29. What are the characteristics of acute diarrhea?

• Most acute diarrhea is the result of an **enteric infection**, viral or bacterial.
• The onset of acute diarrhea is abrupt with a limited duration.
• The focus of the examination is the assessment for **dehydration**.
• If the diarrhea is due to gastroenteritis, the most common cause, the abdomen shows diffuse tenderness and active bowel sounds.
• Focal or rebound tenderness or absent bowel sounds require further radiographic imaging and in many cases laboratory evaluation.

30. Define chronic diarrhea.

The persistence of diarrhea longer than 2 weeks' duration.

31. List the causes of chronic diarrhea by age.

AGE GROUP	CAUSE OF CHRONIC DIARRHEA	
Newborn–3 mo	Postinfection	Short-bowel syndrome
	Protein intolerance	Malnutrition
	Cystic fibrosis	
3 mo–3 yr	Postinfection	Protein intolerance
	Chronic nonspecific diarrhea	Sucrase-isomaltase deficiency
	Giardiasis	Hirschsprung's disease
	Celiac disease	
3–18 yr	Giardiasis	Inflammatory bowel disease
	Celiac disease	Crohn's disease
	Late-onset lactose intolerance	Ulcerative colitis

32. Describe the characteristics of stool infected by various parasites.

CAUSATIVE AGENT	STOOL TYPE	BLOOD IN STOOL	ABDOMINAL PAIN
Rotavirus	Watery, large volume	Rare	Cramps
Giardia	Loose, watery, greasy	Rare	Abdominal distention, cramping
Cryptosporidium	Frequent and watery	Rare	Abdominal pain, weight loss, dehydration
Shigella	Watery, yellow, green with bloody mucus	Yes	Severe pain
Salmonella	Loose, slimy, green	Rare	Moderate pain
Campylobacter	Mucoid, watery, profuse blood	Yes	Severe
Yersinia	Loose green	Occasional	Crampy usually in right lower quadrant
Clostridium difficile	Watery	Yes	Moderate pain

CONTROVERSIES

33. What causes colic?

There are three common theories regarding colic.

1. The crying is due to **abdominal pain**, and the suggested treatment is with medication. The only medication found to work well is **dicyclomine**, which also is found to cause lethargy and sedation. Debate continues as to whether the medicine truly treats abdominal pain or if the sedation diminishes the crying.

2. The infant has an **immature neurologic system** that causes the infant to be extremely sensitive to stimuli, causing unexplained crying. Treatment for colic according to this theory centers on **decreasing** the infant's **stimulation**. One clinical study showed the effectiveness of decreased stimulation on excessive crying.

3. The crying is the infant's attempt to **communicate** needs and wants. Treatment is aimed at the **parents** and helping them interpret the infant's signals more effectively. The infant's cry may indicate that the infant is hungry, is not hungry but wants to suck, wants to be held, is bored and wants stimulation, or is tired and wants to sleep.

34. Discuss the dietary management of children with acute diarrhea.

The use of the **BRAT diet** (*b*ananas, *r*ice cereal, *a*pplesauce, and *t*oast) has been a mainstay treatment for acute diarrhea. More recently the BRAT diet has become controversial. The BRAT diet consists solely of foods containing carbohydrates. It currently is thought that a lot of childhood diarrhea is a result of malabsorption of carbohydrates, and giving an all-carbohydrate diet just increases the diarrhea. Also, a diet of exclusively carbohydrates is unbalanced and provides little energy. The current thought concerning nourishment of children with diarrhea is, in the absence of vomiting, an **age-appropriate diet**, including formula for infants. For older children, chicken with rice soup has been suggested as a reasonable food because it provides fluid, sodium, fat, protein, and rice starch.

BIBLIOGRAPHY

1. Avner JR: Vomiting. In Schwartz MW (ed): Pediatric Primary Care: A Problem-Oriented Approach. St. Louis, Mosby, 1997.
2. Boyle JT: Recurrent abdominal pain: An update. Pediatr Rev 18:310–320, 1997.
3. Bradley RB: Gastroesophageal reflux in children. Adv Nurse Practitioners 9:40, 2001.

4. Castiglia PT: Constipation in children. J Pediatr Health Care 15:200–202, 2001.
5. Gokhale R: Chronic abdominal pain: Inflammatory bowel disease and eosinophilic gastroenteropathy. Pediatr Ann 30:49–55, 2001.
6. Levy J: Gastroesophageal reflux and other causes of abdominal pain. Pediatr Ann 30:42–47, 2001.
7. Melnyk BM: Recurrent pain syndromes in children and adolescents: Unraveling the mystery. Presented at Pediatric Pearls, Children's Hospital, Columbus, OH, 1999.
8. Schwartz MW (ed): Pediatric Primary Care: A Problem-Oriented Approach, 3rd ed. St. Louis, Mosby, 1997.
9. Taubman B: Clinical trial of the treatment of colic by modification of parent-infant interaction. Pediatrics 74:998–1003, 1984.
10. Wong DL: Whaley and Wong's Nursing Care of Infants and Children, 6th ed. St. Louis, Mosby, 1999.
11. Zeiter DK, Hyams JS: Clinical aspects of recurrent abdominal pain. Pediatr Ann 30:17–21, 2001.

11. MUSCULOSKELETAL SYSTEM

Joseann Helmes DeWitt, RN, MSN, C, CLNC

1. **Identify the major developmental milestones involving the musculoskeletal system.**

   Turning over (abdomen to back)   age 5 months
   Crawling   age 9 months
   Walking   age 12–13 months

2. **Name two common congenital birth defects affecting the musculoskeletal system.**
   1. Developmental dysplasia of the hip (DDH)
   2. Clubfoot

3. **Describe DDH.**

   Previously called congenital hip dysplasia, it is an imperfect or abnormal development of the hip, affecting the femoral head, the acetabulum, or both, which results in improper alignment. Incidence is 1–2 in 1000 live births, and it occurs more commonly in females. Of cases, 80% are unilateral, and the disorder affects the left hip three times more often than the right.

4. **List the signs of DDH in the newborn.**
   - Readily apparent at birth
   - Shortening of limb on affected side
   - Unequal gluteal folds
   - Restricted abduction of hip on affected side
   - Positive Ortolani maneuver
   - Positive Barlow maneuver
   - Allis's or Galeazzi's sign

5. **List the signs of DDH in the infant and child.**
   - Trendelenburg's sign
   - Prominent greater trochanter
   - Affected leg shorter than nonaffected leg
   - Marked lordosis
   - Waddling gait
   - Older child with untreated disorder walks with a limp

6. **Describe the Ortolani and Barlow maneuvers.**

   While the child is in a supine position, the knees are brought to midabduction. Forward, then backward pressure is submitted to each hip separately. In the case of dislocation, the femoral head is felt slipping back into the acetabulum (**Ortolani**). An audible click also may be detected. If the femoral head is felt slipping out of position, then slipping back in during this maneuver, the hip is considered dislocatable (**Barlow**). *These maneuvers should be performed only by properly trained and skilled clinicians. An incorrect technique may result in fracture or permanent damage.*

7. **Describe the Trendelenburg sign.**

   The child stands on one foot, then the other; the opposite pelvis dips or tilts downward to maintain erect posture. The pelvis normally tilts upward.

8. Describe the Allis or Galeazzi sign.

Flex the infant's hips and knees at a 90° angle, and assess knee height. The knees are normally the same height. If one knee appears lower than the other, this difference in height indicates hip dislocation.

9. Name three causes of DDH.

1. Genetic predisposition
2. Fetal position in utero
3. Breech delivery

10. Discuss the treatment for DDH.

Treatment begins as soon as DDH is detected and varies according to age and the extent of dysplasia.

- Newborn to age 6 months usually requires application of an external device, such as a **Pavlik harness**, which promotes hip flexion and abduction and prevents hip extension and adduction.
- Children age 6–18 months usually require **skin traction**, followed by reduction, plaster cast, and a brace to maintain abduction.
- For older children, correction often is difficult, and **surgical reduction** is required.

11. Describe the nursing management for a child in a Pavlik harness.

1. Straps must be secure enough to provide hip flexion, without being too tight.
2. The harness is worn continuously for 23 hours per day, removing only to provide hygiene.
3. Prevention of skin breakdown is essential; monitor skin at least twice daily for redness.
4. Teach parents to use only cotton clothing under the harness, *never* to adjust harness without supervision, to avoid powders and lotions, and to monitor skin for redness or breakdown.
5. Straps should be checked and readjusted every 1–2 weeks as scheduled. When the child is in a period of rapid growth, readjustment is necessary to avoid vascular or nerve damage.
6. Discharge planning includes teaching parents to support the hips and buttocks when the infant is out of the harness.

12. What is the expected outcome of treatment for DDH?

The success rate of treatment is higher if DDH is detected in the newborn period than if it is detected when the child is older. Correction becomes more difficult as the child grows, and it is essential that all newborns be screened appropriately for DDH.

13. What is clubfoot?

A congenital birth defect in which the foot is twisted out of the normal shape or position. The overall incidence is 1–2 in 1000 live births, with a higher incidence in males, and 30-50% are bilateral.

14. What causes clubfoot?

The cause is unknown, but theories include a genetic predisposition, intrauterine position, and neuromuscular disorders.

15. How is clubfoot diagnosed?

- Readily apparent at birth
- Radiographs and ultrasonography to assess muscles and bone and the level of severity

16. Discuss the treatment for clubfoot.

Mild forms may be corrected by daily range-of-motion exercises and the use of corrective shoes, such as **Denis-Browne splints**, which are high-top shoes connected by a metal bar. The splint shoes adjust the angle of rotation of the ankle.

More severe forms may require the application of successive **casts** for several days or weeks.

Surgical correction is required between the ages of 4 and 12 months if normal muscle alignment is not attained.

17. Describe the nursing management for a patient with clubfoot.

1. Detection in the newborn period is essential.

2. Teach parents proper use of Denis-Brown shoes and care of the child with a cast to encourage normal growth and development.

3. Teach parents importance of compliance with treatment protocols—outcome depends strongly on compliance with splints, casts, and other treatments.

4. Assess motor development.

5. Postsurgical care includes neurovascular checks every 2 hours for 24 hours, application of ice packs to the foot for 24 hours, elevation of the foot for 24 hours, and pain management.

18. What is the expected outcome of treatment for clubfoot?

Outcome depends on the severity of the deformity. Some deformities respond quickly to treatment, whereas others require prolonged efforts. Even after surgical correction, the child still may have residual deformity but will be able to walk without a limp, run, and play.

19. Describe Legg-Calvé-Perthes disease.

Legg-Calvé-Perthes disease (also called **coxa plana**) is a disorder of the femoral head that causes progressive destruction (necrosis) as a result of interrupted blood supply to the femoral epiphysis. It is an **aseptic necrosis** because no infection is present. It affects children 3–12 years old and is more common in white boys 4–8 years old. Incidence is 1 in 12,000 live births, and it occurs bilaterally in 10–15% of cases.

20. What are the causes of Legg-Calvé-Perthes disease?

Genetic predisposition and mild traumatic injury.

21. List the signs and symptoms of Legg-Calvé-Perthes disease.

• Intermittent appearance of limp on affected side
• Mild pain in hip exacerbated by increased activity and relieved by rest
• Joint dysfunction and limited range of motion
• Stiffness varying from intermittent to constant
• Limb-length inequality
• Pain, soreness, and aching; usually worse on rising or at the end of the day; may be in groin, hip, or knee area
• Tenderness over hip capsule
• External hip rotation (late sign)
• Deterioration of the femoral head on radiograph

22. How is Legg-Calvé-Perthes disease treated?

The goals for all treatment measures are to keep the head of the femur contained in the acetabulum, to promote healing, and to prevent deformity. **Conservative measures**, including traction, braces, leg casts, and leather slings, may require 2–4 years to correct the anomaly. With **surgical correction**, the child resumes normal activities in 3–4 months.

23. Describe the nursing management for Legg-Calvé-Perthes disease.

1. If the patient is on bed rest, monitor for pressure areas, and encourage hobbies that do not require weight bearing.

2. Teach the patient to avoid weight bearing on affected extremity.

3. The child may return to school, and activities that promote achievement of developmental milestones should be encouraged.

4. Educate the child and parents on management and care of brace, skin care, hygiene, and nutrition.

24. What are potential complications of Legg-Calvé-Perthes disease?

The child may experience loss of range of motion and growth disturbances in the affected limb.

25. What is the expected outcome for Legg-Calvé-Perthes disease?

The disease is self-limiting, and the younger the child is when affected, the better the prognosis is for recovery and the natural remodeling of the joint.

26. Define scoliosis.

Scoliosis, the most common spinal deformity, is a lateral S-shaped or C-shaped curvature of the spine. It is seen more often in girls and is most noticeable at the preadolescent growth spurt.

27. Identify causes of scoliosis.

Congenital, idiopathic, and neuromuscular disorders, such as muscular dystrophy or spinal cord trauma.

28. How is scoliosis diagnosed?

- Physical examination
- Radiologic examinations: magnetic resonance imaging, radiographs, bone scans
- Cobb technique (measures degree of curvature)

When assessing for scoliosis, it is important to have the child undressed, and the examiner should view from the posterior aspect.

29. List the signs and symptoms of scoliosis.

- In girls, the hem of skirts does not hang straight.
- Head and hips are not in alignment.
- Asymmetry of rib hump and flank when child bends from waist.
- Prominent scapula.
- Pain generally is not associated with this disorder.

30. List potential complications resulting from scoliosis.

- Loss of flexibility
- Compression of respiratory excursion
- Difficulty with balance and sitting
- Paralysis from compression of nerves

31. Describe the treatment for scoliosis.

The goal of treatment is to stop the progression of the curvature.

- The treatment for **mild curvature** (10–20° curves) is **exercise**. Although exercising does not correct the deformity, it improves posture and strengthens muscles.
- Treatment for **moderate curvature** (20–40° curves) consists of **braces (spinal orthoses)**:
  1. Milwaukee brace—treatment of high thoracic curves (kyphosis). Brace is worn until cessation of bone growth.
  2. Boston brace—treatment of lumbar lordosis
- **Severe curvature** (> 40° curves) requires **spinal straightening and realignment** using rods. Surgical insertion of **instrumentation (internal fixation)** is combined with bone fusion (arthrodesis). Instrumentation used includes:
  1. Harrington instrumentation (posterior instrumentation)
  2. Luque instrumentation (posterior instrumentation)
  3. Dwyer instrumentation (anterior instrumentation)

32. Compare the three methods of spinal rod instrumentation.

	HARRINGTON INSTRUMENTATION	LUQUE INSTRUMENTATION	DWYER INSTRUMENTATION
Surgical approach	Posterior	Posterior	Anterior
Postoperative mobility	Postoperative immobility required. May logroll when permitted	Postoperative immobility *not* required. Maintain head of bed flat for 12 hours; may logroll after 12 hours if permitted. Activity progresses from side lying to sitting, then walking with assistance within a few days	Postoperative immobility required
Postoperative care	Foley catheter to prevent urinary retention, naso-gastric tube, monitor for pain, assess circulation and neurologic status, monitor for paralytic ileus. External molded plastic jacket to be worn to stabilize spine	Foley catheter to prevent urinary retention. Monitor for pain, assess circulation and neurologic status, monitor for paralytic ileus	Foley catheter to prevent urinary retention. Care of thoracotomy incision. Monitor for pain, assess circulation and neurologic status, monitor for paralytic ileus. External molded plastic jacket to be worn to stabilize spine

33. List the general instructions for postoperative insertion of rods.
- Avoid bending or twisting at the waist.
- Do not participate in physical education classes.
- Do not ride horseback, ride a bicycle, or skate.
- Avoid lifting > 10 lb.
- Mild swimming activity is encouraged, but diving should never be attempted.

34. What is osteomyelitis?
Infection of the bone and bone marrow, most often affecting the long bone of the lower extremities. It usually is caused by septicemia, wounds, fractures, burns, or surgery or follows an upper respiratory tract infection. *Staphylococcus* is usually the offending organism affecting older children, and *Haemophilus* is usually the offending organism affecting younger children. Osteomyelitis occurs most commonly in children age 1–12 years and has a higher incidence in boys.

35. List the signs and symptoms of osteomyelitis.
- Acute onset (generally)
- Increased white blood cell count
- Increased erythrocyte sedimentation rate
- Generalized malaise
- Irritability
- Elevated temperature and tachycardia
- Affected site edematous with increased warmth and redness
- Guarding of affected extremity
- Limited range of motion
- Tenderness over affected bone or joint area
- Pain
- Needle aspiration and culture of specimen reveals causative agent

36. Describe the nursing management of osteomyelitis.
   1. Monitor for potential complications.
   2. Administer antibiotics as scheduled—do not skip doses.
   3. Assess the site of infection; monitor for edema, erythema, warmth, or drainage every 4 hours.
   4. Monitor white blood cell count.
   5. Maintain a patent drainage system if present.
   6. Use sterile technique for dressing changes.
   7. Assess for pain, and administer analgesics as prescribed.

37. What is the treatment for osteomyelitis?
   • Intravenous broad-spectrum **antibiotics**—usually high doses, may take for 6 weeks, or change to oral antibiotics
   • **Immobilization** of affected bone or joint
   • **Surgical interventions** to drain abscess

38. List potential complications from osteomyelitis.
   • Abscess
   • Joint or bone damage, especially damage to epiphysis (growth plate)
   • Complications affecting the hepatic, renal, and hematologic systems (related to high dosages of antibiotics)
   • Amputation of affected extremity
   • Interference with growth

39. What is the prognosis for osteomyelitis?
   Prognosis depends on the severity of the infection, rapid identification and treatment, and the general response to the antibiotic therapy.

40. Define muscular dystrophy.
   A group of inherited diseases affecting the muscle, leading to progressive muscular wasting and degeneration of muscle fibers. It is the largest group of muscle diseases affecting children, and it is genetically acquired (X-linked recessive). There are several forms of muscular dystrophy.

41. What is the most severe and most common form of muscular dystrophy?
   Duchenne's or pseudohypertrophic muscular dystrophy.

42. List the signs and symptoms of muscular dystrophy.
   • Generalized muscular weakness and muscle wasting—usually appears during the third year of life (a history of delay in motor development, especially walking, should be investigated further)
   • Difficulty running and climbing stairs
   • Tires easily when walking
   • Waddling gait
   • Lordosis
   • Abnormal gait
   • Frequent falls
   • Gowers' sign
   • As disease progresses, calves, thighs, and upper arms become larger as a result of fatty infiltration (muscle fibers are being replaced with fat [**pseudohypertrophic**])
   • Some mental retardation is common

43. Describe Gowers' sign.
   Gowers' sign, the classic characteristic sign of muscular dystrophy, describes the method in which the hands are used to push up when rising from a squatting or sitting position. The child

begins on the floor, positions himself or herself on the hands and feet, then **pushes** the hands up along the front of the body until he or she achieves a standing position. This is done because the lower extremities are weak, and the child compensates by using the upper extremities.

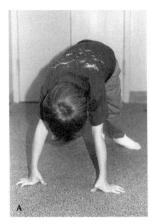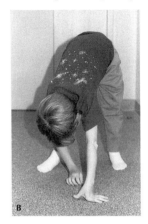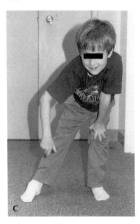

Gowers' sign in a 7-year-old boy with Duchenne's muscular dystrophy. (From McDonald C: Neuromuscular diseases. In Molnar GE, Alexander MA (eds): Pediatric Rehabilitation, 3rd ed. Philadelphia, Hanley & Belfus, 1999, pp 289–330; with permission.)

44. List the methods of diagnosing muscular dystrophy.
Muscle biopsy (identifies presence of fat)
DNA testing
Electromyography
Elevated serum creatine kinase
History and physical findings

45. How is muscular dystrophy treated?
There is no cure for muscular dystrophy. The goal of treatment is to maintain function of unaffected muscles. **Braces** and **surgery** may be necessary. Pharmacologic therapy may include **muscle relaxants** and **glucocorticoids**.

46. Describe the nursing management of a patient with muscular dystrophy.
1. **Respiratory care** is essential. Teach deep breathing and coughing exercises.
2. Teach signs and symptoms of infection.
3. Encourage independence as long as child is capable. Powered wheelchairs, special eating utensils, and other equipment are available.
4. Encourage genetic counseling.
5. Assist family and child in coping with a fatal disease.
6. Teach proper body mechanics and range-of-motion techniques.
7. Refer family to the **Muscular Dystrophy Association** (http://www.mdausa.org/).

47. List potential complications that may occur as a result of muscular dystrophy.
• Atrophy may develop as a result of immobility.
• Contracture deformities may develop as a result of immobility and disease.
• Obesity may result from bed rest and immobility.
• Cardiac complications occur late in disease and may require a pacemaker.
• Infections, especially respiratory, secondary to weak muscles of respiration, occur. Even minor infections require prompt treatment to avoid complications or death.

48. What is the expected outcome for muscular dystrophy?

The disease is progressive, causing gradual muscular wasting. Usually the child is unable to walk by the age of 12. The terminal stage usually involves the diaphragm and the muscles of respiration. Death often results from respiratory tract infection or cardiac failure.

49. Define juvenile rheumatoid arthritis.

A chronic inflammatory disease affecting the synovium of the joints. The cause is unknown; however, it is linked to infectious and autoimmune disorders. It has a tendency to occur most often in young children (ages 2–5) and in prepubertal children (ages 9–12) and affects girls more often than boys.

50. List the signs and symptoms of juvenile rheumatoid arthritis.

Tenderness	Pain may or may not be present
Warm to touch, may have fever	Morning stiffness or stiffness after inactivity
Loss of motion or limited motion	Limp
Stiffness and swelling	

51. How is juvenile rheumatoid arthritis diagnosed?

There is no specific diagnostic test, but rheumatoid factor and antinuclear antibody tests may be positive.

52. What is the treatment for juvenile rheumatoid arthritis?

The primary goal is to preserve mobility and prevent loss of joint function.
- Range-of-motion exercises—best performed in the bath or pool. Warm water can help relax muscles and reduce stiffness
- Splints or sandbags to maintain alignment
- Physical and occupational therapy
- Application of heat—paraffin baths, warm baths, warm compresses
- Pharmacologic therapy—salicylates, nonsteroidal anti-inflammatory agents, corticosteroids, aspirin, cytotoxic agents, analgesics

53. Describe the nursing management for juvenile rheumatoid arthritis.

1. Teach the patient and family methods to reduce pain and early morning stiffness, such as a warm shower or soak in the morning before beginning activities.
2. Maintain proper body alignment.
3. Maintain splints.
4. Administer analgesics and anti-inflammatory medications before beginning therapy and exercises.
5. Teach proper active and passive range-of-motion exercise.
6. Encourage normal activities and routines as much as possible
7. Use warm compresses.
8. Teach adequate nutrition and fluid intake.

54. Name the most common causes of fractures in the pediatric population.

Birth trauma
Injury/trauma (motor vehicle accidents, sports injuries)
Child abuse

55. What are the most common types of fractures seen in the pediatric population?

- Fractures of the forearm—the child extends the hand to break the fall and may break fingers, wrist, elbow, and shoulder
- Clavicle fractures sustained during birth
- Femoral neck fractures—result of motor vehicle crash
- Knee fractures in adolescents—result of sports injuries

*Hip fractures are **rare** in the pediatric population, and **abuse** should be suspected until a cause is verified.*

56. List the clinical manifestations of fracture in the child.
Pain and tenderness
Generalized swelling
Crepitus
Immobility or decreased range of motion
Ecchymosis
Suspect a fracture in a young child who refuses to walk.

57. What is the most common diagnostic tool used for identifying fractures?
Radiograph. A comparison between a radiograph of the affected extremity and one of the unaffected extremity should be done.

58. When should physical abuse be suspected based on radiographs?
Abuse should be suspected when radiographs of children reveal fractures at various stages of healing. In abuse of infants, radiographs reveal **periosteal bleeding** in the long bones as the result of twisting, pulling, and rough handling. This bleeding is not evident until 3–6 weeks after the injury occurred.

59. Describe the nursing management of a child with fracture.
1. Be alert for the signs and symptoms of fractures in children: pain, tenderness, swelling, crepitus.
2. Monitor for pain and provide analgesics as prescribed.
3. Promote mobility.
4. Provide cast care, traction care, and postoperative care as needed.
5. Monitor for vascular compromise.

60. What are the five P's in assessment of circulatory impairment?
Pain   Pulselessness   Paralysis
Pallor   Paresthesia

61. Describe the nursing management of a child in traction.
1. Monitor for appropriate alignment, and ensure that weights hang freely.
2. Maintain skin integrity.
3. Promote pulmonary hygiene.
4. Promote adequate fluid and fiber intake to prevent constipation.
5. Provide stimulation appropriate for developmental age to promote growth and development.
6. Encourage limited mobility as permitted.
7. Encourage parents to hold child.
8. Avoid pressure on the popliteal space to prevent nerve damage.
9. Provide adequate pain relief.

62. Which sports that have the highest rates of injuries for the pediatric population?
Gymnastics
Football
Ice hockey

63. Describe nursing measures for prevention of sports injuries in the pediatric population.
1. Encourage parents of all children participating in sports activities to ensure the child has a thorough medical screening and evaluation before allowing him or her to participate in sports activities.

2. Encourage the correct training and conditioning of children participating in sports activities.

3. Encourage the use of protective equipment (i.e., helmets, goggles, and pads).

4. Provide first-aid training for coaches and parents, and inform them that most sports injuries occur during the practice sessions rather than the games.

5. Educate parents and coaches that the child's participation in sports should be based on physical maturity, height, weight, and skills. Participation should not be based on age.

6. Educate parents that the American Academy of Pediatrics opposes pediatric participation in boxing and the use of trampolines.

BIBLIOGRAPHY

1. Ball J, Bindler R: Pediatric Nursing: Caring for Children, 2nd ed. Stamford, CT, Appleton & Lange, 1999, pp 819–861.
2. McKinney ES, Ashwill JW, Murray SS, et al: Maternal-Child Nursing. Philadelphia, W.B. Saunders, 2000, pp 1384–1429.
3. Pillitteri A: Child Health Nursing: Care of the Child and Family. Philadelphia, Lippincott, 1999, pp 1485–1520.
4. Wong DL: Whaley and Wong's Nursing Care of Infants and Children, 6th ed. St. Louis, Mosby, 1999, pp 1487–2001.

12. GENITOURINARY SYSTEM

Joseann Helmes DeWitt, RN, MSN, C, CLNC

1. What is the normal bladder capacity of children?
Infants: 60 mL
Toddlers: 285–400 mL
School-age children: 840–1000 mL

2. At what age do children normally achieve urinary continence?
Daytime: 2.5–3 years
Nighttime: 4–5 years

3. Name three congenital birth defects affecting the genitourinary system.
Hypospadias
Epispadias
Exstrophy of the bladder (externalization of bladder)

4. Define hypospadias and epispadias.
Hypospadias is a congenital birth defect whereby the urinary meatus in the male is located on the ventral (underside) aspect of the penis rather than on the end of the penis. This defect occurs in varying degrees, from just below the tip of the penis in mild forms to severe forms located on the scrotum. In **epispadias**, the urethral opening is located on the dorsal (top) aspect of the penis. This defect is much rarer than hypospadias. These disorders are detected readily on the newborn assessment.

5. What is the treatment for hypospadias and epispadias?
For defects requiring **surgical intervention**, the optimal time for repair is between ages 6 and 18 months, before the child has mutilation fears. Surgical correction may be simple or complex and may require staging.

6. Describe nursing interventions for hypospadias and epispadias.
1. Teach the family to avoid circumcision because the skin may be needed in the future for use during surgical reconstruction.
2. Teach the family preoperative and postoperative care.
3. Support the family and address psychosocial needs.

7. Summarize the postoperative care for hypospadias and epispadias.
• Inform parents and child that the penis will be bound in a pressure dressing.
• If the child is older, explain to him that the penis is still there.
• Catheter or stint remains in place for at least 10 days to allow the new urethra to heal.
• *Never* clamp catheter; this can result in trauma to the new urethra.
• Assess for pain and provide analgesics as indicated.

8. What home care instructions should be provided to the family for postoperative care of hypospadias or epispadias?
1. Do not allow child to play in sand or dirt.
2. Do not allow child to straddle or play on riding toys.
3. Do not allow child to engage in rough play.
4. Avoid tub bathing—sponge bathing is recommended until stint is removed.

5. Educate family to recognize signs and symptoms of urinary tract infection (UTI) and to report suspected complications.

6. Encourage adequate fluid intake to promote urinary output.

9. Define phimosis.

A narrowing (**stenosis**) of the opening of the foreskin. It is a normal finding in boys younger than 3 years old and usually resolves without incident. If it does not resolve, complications from constriction occur.

10. List the signs and symptoms of phimosis.

Dysuria (pain)	Urinary stream diverted to side
Hematuria	Recurrent infections
Decreased urinary stream	Irritation
Tender foreskin	

11. How is phimosis treated?

Gradual **retraction of foreskin** is performed several times a day to stretch gently the tight foreskin. *Always replace the foreskin after stretching.* A **circumcision** is performed to remove foreskin if phimosis is severe.

12. What severe complication can result from phimosis?

Paraphimosis, a medical emergency, results from constriction of the tight band of foreskin, which obstructs the blood supply to the penis. Immediate intervention is required to prevent irreversible damage.

13. Define cryptorchidism.

Cryptorchidism (undescended testicles) is the failure of one or both testes to descend normally into the scrotum. It occurs more frequently in premature infants because testes normally descend during the seventh to ninth month of gestation.

14. Identify assessments performed to determine the presence of cryptorchidism.

- Manual examination of scrotal contents should be performed during the first 2 years of life—one or both testes may be undescended.
- Affected side appears empty, not full.
- No rugae (wrinkles) are present.
- Sac is empty to palpation.

15. What potential complications can occur from untreated cryptorchidism?

Infertility from body heat destroying sperm
More prone to testicular tumors
Testicular torsion
Psychological effects of defect

16. Describe the management of cryptorchidism.

Of cases of cryptorchidism, 80% correct spontaneously by the age of 1 year. If spontaneous descent does not occur, an **orchiopexy**, the surgical correction procedure, is performed between ages 1 and 2 years. Other treatment options include the administration of luteinizing hormones and human chorionic gonadotropic hormones to attempt to stimulate descent.

17. Define testicular torsion.

Testicular torsion is the twisting of the testicle on the spermatic cord. This results in loss of blood supply to the testicle and epididymis and other structures. It occurs most frequently in boys age 10–14 years, following a trauma during sports activities, but it can occur at any age. Testicular torsion is considered a surgical emergency; early recognition is essential.

18. **List signs and symptoms of testicular torsion.**
    Sudden onset of unilateral pain, radiating to groin area
    Abdominal pain
    Nausea and vomiting
    Tender scrotum

19. **What is the treatment and outcome of testicular torsion?**
    Surgical correction to restore circulation and prevent irreparable testicular damage. Recovery usually is uneventful.

20. **Define nocturnal enuresis and diurnal enuresis.**
    Nocturnal enuresis, commonly called **bedwetting**, is involuntary voiding after the age of 4 or 5. **Diurnal enuresis** is daytime wetting in a child who is old enough to maintain bladder control.

21. **Define primary and secondary enuresis.**
    Primary enuresis—a child has never achieved complete bladder control.
    Secondary enuresis—a child has achieved a period of bladder control.

22. **What procedures typically are performed to determine or rule out the cause of enuresis?**
    • Urinalysis and urine culture to rule out UTI (most common cause)
    • Radiologic studies (intravenous pyelogram, voiding cystourethrogram, and sonograms) to rule out mass, obstruction, or disorder of urinary structures
    • Physical examination to rule out constipation or fecal impaction
    • Serum laboratory studies to rule out diabetes mellitus and diabetes insipidus
    If all other causes are ruled out, consider a psychological cause

23. **How is enuresis managed?**
    • Some cases resolve spontaneously, depending on the underlying cause.
    • Conditioning alarms, awakening the child during the night to void, restricting fluids after 5 P.M., and encouraging frequent toileting during the day have proved effective, although relapses tend to occur.
    • Pharmacologic options include imipramine (Tofranil), oxybutynin, and desmopressin (DDAVP). Relapses also occur after treatment with pharmacologic agents.
    • Parental education is important. Encourage parents not to punish, shame, or scold the child.
    • The parents and child need emotional support.

24. **Identify common predisposing factors of UTIs in children.**
    • Urinary stasis (number one predisposing factor)
    • Occurs more commonly in girls because of short urethra and close proximity of urethra to meatus
    • Poor hygiene
    • Uncircumcised penis
    • Use of antibiotics
    • Sexual activity (especially in girls)
    • Functional obstruction

25. **List the clinical manifestations of UTIs in children younger than age 2.**
    • Signs and symptoms often nonspecific
    • Frequent or infrequent voiding
    • Strong urine odor
    • Gastrointestinal symptoms, such as difficulty feeding, diarrhea, and vomiting

- Cries when voids
- Diaper rash

26. List the clinical manifestations of UTIs in older children.

Enuresis	Costovertebral tenderness
Strong urine odor	Hematuria
Fever and chills	Mild abdominal pain
Frequency and urgency	High fever, vomiting, malaise (as infection progresses)
Dysuria	

Approximately 40% of all UTIs in children are **asymptomatic** and are discovered incidentally.

27. How is the diagnosis of urinary tract infection made?
Urine culture and urinalysis.

28. List common offending organisms in UTI.

E. coli (most common causative agent)	*Staphylococcus aureus*
Enterobacter	*Proteus*
Enterococcus	*Pseudomonas*
Klebsiella	

29. What are the findings of urinalysis in UTI?
1. Positive for red blood cells and white blood cells
2. Positive for protein

30. Describe the management for UTIs.
- Antibiotic therapy—educate parents to administer the full course of antibiotics as prescribed.
- Increase fluid intake.
- Monitor intake and output.
- Educate parents and child in proper hygiene, frequent voiding, avoiding bubble baths (causes irritation), and use of cotton panties in girls.
- If child has frequent UTIs, further investigation is warranted.
- Assess for sexual abuse or sexual activity.
- Follow-up urine cultures must be performed to determine successful treatment and to detect recurrence.
- Encourage the toilet-trained child to void at least four times a day and to avoid holding urine.

31. Why is antibiotic treatment of UTI essential?
To avoid spread of bacteria to kidneys (pyelonephritis).

32. Define acute poststreptococcal glomerulonephritis.
Also called **acute glomerulonephritis**, acute poststreptococcal glomerulonephritis refers to a group of disorders characterized by inflammation of the glomeruli of the kidney. It occurs as an autoimmune response to a previous streptococcal infection affecting another body system (respiratory tract, skin). It affects boys most often and occurs most commonly between ages 5 and 10 years.

33. What causes acute poststreptococcal glomerulonephritis?
The most common cause is **poststreptococcal infection**, usually from group A beta-hemolytic streptococcal infection of the respiratory tract (**streptococcal pharyngitis**) or of the skin (**streptococcal impetigo**). The symptoms appear approximately 10 days after the infection.

34. **List the signs and symptoms of acute poststreptococcal glomerulonephritis.**
   - Initial onset of gross hematuria and mild proteinuria (0+ to 2+)
   - Oliguria (reduced urine volume)
   - Periorbital edema
   - Edema of face, abdomen, and lymph nodes
   - Pallor, lethargy, irritability, and headache
   - Abdominal pain, anorexia, and vomiting
   - Dysuria
   - Urine appears cloudy and brown (cola or tea colored)
   - Fatigue
   - Elevated blood pressure ranging from mild to moderate to severe

35. **How is acute poststreptococcal glomerulonephritis diagnosed?**
   - Urinalysis shows hematuria, proteinuria (0+ to 2+), and increased specific gravity.
   - Elevated blood urea nitrogen and creatinine may be present.
   - Electrolytes are normal unless renal failure is present.
   - Anemia is present as a result of hemodilution.
   - Streptozyme test is positive.
   - Urine cultures are negative.

36. **Describe the expected clinical course of acute poststreptococcal glomerulonephritis.**
   - **Acute phase** includes the clinical manifestations and typically lasts 4-10 days but can last 2-3 weeks.
   - **Diuresis**, the first sign of improvement, occurs in massive amounts. The edema subsides, the patient begins to feel better, blood pressure improves, and gross hematuria is no longer present, but microscopic hematuria is present for several months.
   - **Convalescence** follows the diuresis phase; it can take weeks to months for the patient to recover fully.

37. **Discuss the pharmacologic management for acute poststreptococcal glomerulonephritis.**
   - Antihypertensive agents to control blood pressure
   - Diuretics (furosemide [Lasix]) to promote diuresis (some consider diuretics to have little value in treatment of acute glomerulonephritis)
   - Corticosteroids to decrease the inflammatory response
   - Penicillin to ensure eradication of streptococcal infection

38. **Are antibiotics needed for treatment of acute glomerulonephritis?**
   No. This is not an active infection but is the result of an antigen-antibody response to a past infection.

39. **Summarize the nutritional management for acute poststreptococcal glomerulonephritis.**
   The degree of dietary restrictions is determined by the severity of the edema present.
   Sodium restrictions include no added salt, and avoid foods high in sodium. Mild sodium restriction may be necessary, depending on edema.
   Potassium restrictions are needed especially during the oliguric phase. Avoid foods high in potassium.
   Protein usually is not restricted.
   Fluid restriction usually is not necessary unless oliguric.

40. **Discuss nursing management for acute poststreptococcal glomerulonephritis.**
   If blood pressure and urine output are normal, the patient can be treated at home. Parental education to identify complications is essential. Hospitalization is necessary in

presence of edema, hypertension, and gross hematuria. Nursing interventions during hospitalization include:
- Monitoring blood pressure every 1–2 hours during the acute phase, then every 4 hours
- Seizure precautions
- Monitoring fluid volume status every 1–2 hours (urine output should equal 1–2 mL/kg/hr)
- Daily weights
- Administration of antihypertensive agents and other medications as indicated
- Assessment of neurologic status every 2–4 hours
- Measures to prevent skin breakdown in the presence of edema (e.g., reposition every 2 hours, elevate extremities, support scrotum)
- Maintain bed in semi-Fowler's position
- Assessment for increasing respiratory difficulty

Bed rest is not necessary, but limit activity until kidney function returns to normal.

41. List potential complications that may result from acute poststreptococcal glomerulonephritis.
- Encephalopathy as a result of hypertension
- Cardiac decompensation as a result of excess fluid volume
- Pulmonary edema and liver enlargement
- Skin breakdown as a result of edema
- Acute renal failure if oliguria progresses to anuria (rare)
- Chronic renal disease

42. What is the expected outcome after treatment of acute poststreptococcal glomerulonephritis?
Recovery is spontaneous. The course of illness ranges from 1 to 2 weeks and usually requires only a short hospital stay. Although prognosis is excellent and most children recover completely, a small percentage (< 2%) develop chronic nephritis.

43. Define nephrotic syndrome.
Nephrotic syndrome (also called **nephrosis**) refers to a disorder of the kidney characterized by altered glomeruli permeability, which leads to massive loss of protein in the urine. Males are affected more often, and it occurs primarily in preschool children, peaking at age 2–3 years, but it can occur at any age. There are several types.

44. What is the most common type of nephrotic syndrome?
Minimal change nephrotic syndrome occurs in 80% of the cases.

45. What is the cause of nephrotic syndrome?
The cause is unknown. It is believed, however, to be an autoimmune response resulting from an antigen-antibody reaction. Nephrotic syndrome often follows a viral upper respiratory infection, although this seems to be a precipitating factor rather than a causative factor.

46. List the signs and symptoms of nephrotic syndrome.
- Proteinuria (3+ to 4+), edema, hypoalbuminemia, and hyperlipidemia are the four classic signs.
- Insidious weight gain—occurs gradually over days to weeks
- Shifting edema. Morning periorbital and sacral edema shifts to scrotal and labial edema and ascites during the day. It progresses to massive edema
- Oliguria
- Urine dark, frothy, and opalescent
- Extreme pallor

- Blood pressure normal or slightly low
- Irritable, easily fatigued
- Muercke lines on nails resulting from hypoalbuminemia

47. Summarize the laboratory values used to diagnose nephrotic syndrome.
- Urinalysis reveals massive proteinuria, casts, and increased specific gravity.
- Gross hematuria usually does not occur.
- Serum laboratory values indicate hypoalbuminemia and hyperlipidemia.
- Platelet count may be elevated as a result of hemoconcentration.
- Hemoglobin and hematocrit usually are normal or elevated.
- Hyponatremia is present.
- Renal biopsy specimen shows a normal-appearing kidney.
- Elevated erythrocyte sedimentation rate is present.
- Electrolytes usually are normal.

48. List the pharmacologic agents for management for nephrotic syndrome.
Prednisone—the mainstay of therapy, to suppress the autoimmune response (may take for 2 weeks to several months)
Cyclophosphamide (Cytoxan)—may be administered in conjunction with prednisone if the child fails to respond to steroids
Spironolactone, furosemide, and **hydrochlorothiazide**—may be used to treat severe edema but should be used with caution to prevent hypovolemia
Broad-spectrum antimicrobials—to reduce risk of infection
Albumin—to correct hypoalbuminemia temporarily

49. Summarize the nutritional management for nephrotic syndrome.
- Dietary management usually is limited to no added salt; other restrictions are rare.
- The child generally has a poor appetite, and measures are necessary to prevent malnutrition.
- Consuming extra protein has not been shown to improve hypoalbuminemia, although some recommend encouraging a diet high in protein.
- Fluid intake usually is not restricted unless it is necessary during the acute phase.
- Encouraging foods high in potassium is necessary, especially during the administration of diuretics.

50. List nursing management tasks for nephrotic syndrome.
1. Provide meticulous skin care to edematous skin.
2. Avoid intramuscular injections.
3. Maintain elevated head of bed to reduce periorbital edema.
4. Reposition frequently, and provide scrotal support if necessary.
5. Encourage small, frequent meals.
6. Monitor intake and output, vital signs, and daily weight.
7. Measure abdominal girth.
8. Maintain bed rest to conserve energy.
9. Instruct to avoid contact with persons with infection.
10. Maintain bed in semi-Fowler's position.
11. Teach parents to test urine for protein with a dipstick.

51. List potential complications that may result from nephrotic syndrome.
- Edema, leading to skin breakdown
- Poor nutritional intake secondary to anorexia from ascites, leading to malnourishment
- Potential for hypertension, but generally blood pressure is normal to low
- Potential for infection related to immunosuppression
- Difficulty breathing as a result of ascites

52. What is the expected outcome from treatment of nephrotic syndrome?

This is a self-limiting disease, and the prognosis is usually good. If the patient responds well to treatment, renal function should return to normal or near-normal. Of patients, 50% may relapse 5 years later, and 20% may relapse 10 years later.

53. Compare acute poststreptococcal glomerulonephritis and nephrotic syndrome.

MANIFESTATIONS AND TREATMENT	ACUTE POSTSTREPTOCOCCAL GLOMERULONEPHRITIS	NEPHROTIC SYNDROME
Causative agent	Autoimmune response to a previous streptococcal infection	Exact cause is unknown; believed to be an autoimmune response of an antigen-antibody reaction
Peak age at onset	5–7 yr	2–3 yr
Hematuria	Microscopic or gross	Microscopic or none
Proteinuria	Mild-to-moderate (0+ to 2+)	Massive (3+ to 4+)
Hypoalbuminemia (low serum protein levels)	Normal or slightly decreased	Markedly decreased
Edema	Generally periorbital and peripheral	Severe generalized edema
Blood pressure	Elevated	Normal or slightly decreased
Nutritional restrictions		
Sodium	Depends on the severity of edema	No added salt
Protein	Not restricted unless oliguric	Not restricted
Potassium	Avoid foods high in potassium	Encourage foods high in potassium if receiving diuretics
Fluid restrictions	Usually not restricted unless oliguric	Fluid restriction usually not necessary unless in acute phase
Treatment	No specific treatment, usually supportive. Blood pressure control. Possible use of diuretics. Corticosteroids	Prednisone, spironolactone, furosemide, hydrochlorothiazide, albumin
Recovery	Usually spontaneous with complete recovery. A small percentage may develop chronic nephritis	Self-limiting disease. Prognosis good but may relapse 5–10 yr later

BIBLIOGRAPHY

1. Ball J, Bindler R: Pediatric Nursing: Caring for Children, 2nd ed. Stamford, CT, Appleton & Lange, 1999, pp 660–709.
2. Hogg RJ, Portman RJ, Milliner D, et al: Evaluation and management of proteinuria and nephrotic syndrome in children: Recommendations from a pediatric nephrology panel established at the National Kidney Foundation conference on proteinuria. Pediatrics 105:1242–1249, 2000.
3. McKinney ES, Ashwill JW, Murray SS, et al: Maternal-Child Nursing. Philadelphia, W.B. Saunders, 2000, pp 1159–1190.
4. Pillitteri A: Child Health Nursing: Care of the Child and Family. Philadelphia, Lippincott, 1999, pp 770–801.
5. Wong DL: Whaley and Wong's Nursing Care of Infants and Children, 6th ed. St. Louis, Mosby, 1999.

13. PEDIATRIC ONCOLOGY

Karen Wolownik, RNC, MSN, CPNP

1. Name the most common malignancies of childhood.

Leukemia (>30%)

Central nervous system (CNS) tumors (> 20%)

Lymphomas (> 10%)

2. What is the incidence of acute lymphoblastic leukemia (ALL)?

ALL affects approximately 2500–3000 children each year in the United States.

3. Describe factors that may predispose children develop ALL.

Genetic factors are presumed to play a significant role in the cause of acute leukemias, as shown by the occurrence of familial leukemia, the high incidence of leukemia in identical twins, and the association between various chromosomal abnormalities and childhood ALL. Children with trisomy 21, or **Down's syndrome**, are 15 times more likely to develop leukemia than normal children.

Environmental factors, such as exposure to ionizing radiation and certain toxic chemicals, can facilitate the development of acute leukemia.

Some reports suggest there is an increased risk for ALL in children who have had recent **viral infections** or who were born to mothers with viral infections.

Children with various congenital **immunodeficiency diseases** have an increased risk of developing lymphoid malignancies, as do patients receiving long-term treatment with **immunosuppressive drugs**.

4. Discuss the role of CNS prophylaxis in ALL.

CNS relapse is of particular concern for children with leukemia because it constitutes a major obstacle to overall treatment success. The CNS acts as a sanctuary site in which leukemic cells are protected by the blood-brain barrier from therapeutic amounts of systemically infused chemotherapeutic agents.

CNS prophylaxis is given by **intrathecal chemotherapy** or **cranial irradiation** or both. This preventive therapy may be associated with acute or subacute neurotoxic effects. **Methotrexate**, a chemotherapy agent used often for intrathecal administration, may be associated with acute arachnoiditis.

5. What do nurses need to be aware of to care for patients receiving CNS prophylaxis?

1. Nurses should monitor carefully for headaches, nausea and vomiting, meningism, and other signs of **increased intracranial pressure** occurring 12–24 hours after **intrathecal therapy**. These reactions usually are self-limited and not severe, but they can be of particular concern for patients and families.

2. **Cranial radiation** may cause **somnolence syndrome**. Somnolence syndrome occurs typically 5–7 weeks after radiation and is characterized by somnolence, lethargy, anorexia, fever, and irritability. The nurse should reassure the patient and family that this condition usually is temporary and should resolve in 1–3 weeks.

6. What is the most common renal malignancy of childhood?

Wilms' tumor.

7. How do patients typically present with Wilms' tumor?

Wilms' tumor typically presents as abdominal swelling or the presence of an abdominal mass. Parents often notice the abdominal enlargement while bathing or dressing the child.

8. List other frequent findings in Wilms' tumor.
Abdominal pain
Gross hematuria
Fever

9. What is the treatment for Wilms' tumor?
A combined-modality approach is the basis for treatment. All patients have **surgical removal** (complete or partial nephrectomy) of the tumor (if possible), then receive **chemotherapy** or **radiation therapy** or both. Therapy is determined based on the stage of the disease (stage I to IV) and histology (favorable vs. unfavorable).

10. List the chemotherapy agents used in most regimens for Wilms' tumor.
Vincristine
Actinomycin D
Doxorubicin
Cyclophosphamide

11. Describe the nursing care for patients after surgical removal of Wilms' tumor.

NURSING DIAGNOSIS	NURSING ASSESSMENT AND INTERVENTION
Alteration in elimination	Maintain patency of Foley catheter Check urine output every 2 hr; should be 2 ml/kg/hr Perform urine dipstick and maintain specific gravity ≤ 1.010 Administer IV hydration Monitor serum electrolytes
Alteration in fluid volume excess	Measure urine output every 2 hr and keep accurate records of intake and output Monitor BP and pulse every 2 hr for hypertension and tachycardia Auscultate lung sounds for presence of rales or crackles Perform daily weights Administer diuretics as indicated Monitor serum electrolytes daily; note BUN, creatinine, potassium, and sodium
Alteration in comfort	Position for comfort Administer narcotics every 2–3 hr or as needed. If pain remains uncontrolled, consider use of patient-controlled analgesia Administer nonsteroidal antiinflammatory drugs around the clock to provide synergy
Potential for infection	Administer prophylactic antibiotics Monitor WBC count Use aseptic technique in the care of all catheters and central and peripheral lines Perform thorough hand washing Cleanse Foley catheter and urethral meatus with soap and water every 8 hr Promote effective breathing patterns by encouraging use of incentive spirometry, coughing and deep breathing, and turning and positioning every 2 hr Inspect incision site daily for signs of infection (erythema, exudate) and close wound approximation Maintain sterile wound dressings Provide adequate nutrition

BP, blood pressure; BUN, blood urea nitrogen; WBC, white blood cell.

12. What is Hodgkin's disease?

A malignancy that arises in the lymph nodes. The cause is unknown, although there may be a viral association with Epstein-Barr virus.

13. How is Hodgkin's disease diagnosed?
- History
- Physical examination with measurement of enlarged lymph nodes
- Complete blood count with differential, erythrocyte sedimentation rate, renal and hepatic function tests, and alkaline phosphatase level
- Lymph node biopsy
- Thoracic, abdominal, and pelvic computed tomography scan or magnetic resonance imaging
- Gallium or positron emission tomography scan
- Bone marrow biopsy
- Bone scan

14. Discuss the future trends in treatment of Hodgkin's disease.

Monoclonal antibodies and **targeted cellular immunotherapy** are being explored in an effort to reduce disease burden and decrease relapse rate. **Allogeneic stem cell transplant** is being explored for patients with relapsed or refractory Hodgkin's disease. After high-dose therapy, patients receive low-dose chemotherapy and immunosuppression followed by infusion of donor stem cells. The goal in this therapy is to reduce toxicities associated with high-dose chemotherapy but provide enough immunosuppression to allow the donor cells to grow. When the donor cells engraft, they show a graft-versus-tumor effect that, it is hoped, will allow patients to remain in a complete remission and reduce relapse rates. Although this is still a novel approach, early studies have shown it to have great potential for improving outcome in high-risk patients.

15. List nursing interventions that can help lessen the pediatric oncology patient's anxiety and facilitate coping with invasive procedures.

1. Teach coping strategies that can be used during the procedure to give the child a sense of control and focus (i.e., imagery and deep breathing).

2. Provide age-appropriate information regarding the procedure the child will undergo.

3. Use medical play to teach the child about the procedure.

4. Ensure that all information is honest and accurate, even if it is unpleasant, to foster trust.

5. Attempt to prepare the child but do not force preparation on the child because some children avoid information and would rather not know.

6. Introduce patients and families to other patients who have had similar experiences.

16. What are the three phases of standard chemotherapy regimens and what are the goals in each?

CHEMOTHERAPY PHASE	WHEN INSTITUTED	GOALS
Induction	Initial therapy	To eliminate as many cancer cells as possible To obtain a complete remission
Consolidation	Given after remission is complete	To ensure complete eradication of disease
Maintenance	Given for several months to years after consolidation, depending on disease	To maintain a complete remission To minimize late effects To prevent drug resistance from developing

17. What is intensification?

If higher doses of chemotherapy are used during consolidation than induction, the therapy is called intensification (often given in **acute myeloid leukemia**).

18. Define tumor lysis syndrome (TLS).

TLS occurs when a large number of tumor cells are destroyed quickly in response to chemotherapy or radiotherapy. Onset usually is rapid and occurs within 24–72 hours of initiation of chemotherapy. When tumor cells die, nucleic acids and intracellular metabolites (potassium and phosphorus) are released and exceed the excretory capacity of the kidneys. The nucleic acids are converted to uric acid in the liver and may crystallize leading to obstruction of the kidneys and acute renal failure.

19. What are the signs and symptoms of TLS?

Clinical manifestations are related to the associated electrolyte imbalances:

Hyperkalemia
Arrhythmias
Muscle weakness and paresthesia
Nausea
Diarrhea
Abdominal cramps
Hypocalcemia
Muscle cramps and twitching
Tetany
Confusion
Convulsions
Hyperphosphatemia
Anuria
Oliguria
Azotemia

If TLS is not adequately controlled and the patient develops **acute renal failure with fluid overload**, additional manifestations may include:
Decreased urine output
Increased weight gain
Hypertension
Pulmonary or peripheral edema

20. List nursing assessments and interventions that may prevent TLS.

1. Assess weight, intake and output, and response to diuretics. Monitor for signs of fluid overload.

2. Assess serum electrolytes every 12 hours or as indicated. Observe for signs of hyperkalemia, hypocalcemia, and hyperphosphatemia.

21. Describe treatment of TLS.

Treatment is aimed at management of metabolic disturbances and supportive care.
- Correct fluid and electrolyte imbalances with diuretics; sodium polystyrene sulfonate (Kayexalate) for hyperkalemia; aluminum hydroxide gel (Amphojel) for hyperphosphatemia; oral or intravenous calcium supplementation; and allopurinol, a xanthine oxidase inhibitor, to decrease uric acid formation.
- Administer intravenous hydration and alkalization (with intravenous sodium bicarbonate).
- Monitor strict intake and output.
- Perform dipstick urine test for specific gravity (< 1.010) and pH (> 7.0).
- Prepare patients for the possibility of temporary hemodialysis if kidney damage is severe.

22. Define neutropenia.

A reduction of circulating neutrophils (mature white blood cells) that can be defined as an **absolute neutrophil count** (ANC) of < 1000/mm^3.

23. How is the ANC measured?

By multiplying the percentage of granulocytes (neutrophils and bands) by the WBC count.

24. Explain the significance of neutropenia.

The degree of neutropenia may vary among patients and therapeutic regimens. More important than the degree of neutropenia is the **duration** of it. The risk of infection is much higher during periods of **prolonged neutropenia** (> 14 days) with a higher ANC than during shorter periods with a lower ANC.

25. List the general guidelines that should be implemented to prevent infection in neutropenic patients.

Hand washing is the most important and effective procedure for preventing nosocomial infection.

Visitors should be limited during periods of prolonged or severe neutropenia to lessen exposure to infectious organisms.

Use of masks varies from institution to institution but routinely does not reduce the occurrence of nosocomial infection significantly. Visitors or health care workers with transmissible respiratory illness should not come in contact with the patient, but if contact is necessary, they should wear a mask.

Use of prophylactic antibiotics varies from institution to institution. Antibiotics should be used carefully to reduce the development of drug-resistant pathogens.

Airflow in patient rooms should be positive pressure (i.e., air flows from inside the room to the hall or out through a vent).

Plants and dried or fresh flowers should not be allowed in the rooms because *Aspergillus* have been isolated from the soil of potted ornamental plants and the surface of dried flower arrangements and fresh flowers.

26. What should be done if a neutropenic patient develops a fever?

1. Appropriate **cultures** should be obtained: blood (from all lumina of the venous access device), urine, throat, and stool (especially *Clostridium difficile*).

2. A **chest radiograph** should be obtained if signs or symptoms of lung involvement are present.

3. **Antibiotics** should be started within 1 hour of onset of fever. Initially, broad-spectrum antibiotics to cover gram-positive and gram-negative organisms are started. If fever or signs of infection persist and blood cultures remain negative after 48–72 hours on antibiotics, a prophylactic **antifungal** agent may be added until all blood cultures are final, which may take 7–10 days.

4. A **complete physical examination** should be performed, including assessment for perianal pain or inflammation; mucositis or oral ulcers; severe abdominal tenderness or cramping; and erythema, drainage, or edema of any intravenous sites or wounds.

5. **Vital signs** should be assessed for increase or decrease in temperature, increased heart rate, or increased respirations.

6. **Monitor** for:
   Change in level of consciousness
   Decrease in urine output
   Increase serum glucose or glucosuria

27. How do you know when an oncology patient requires a packed red blood cell transfusion?

There is no absolute hemoglobin or hematocrit level to indicate when a patient requires a transfusion. In general, most oncology patients receive a packed red blood cell transfusion if the serum hemoglobin is ≤ 8.0 g/dL or the hematocrit is ≤ 25 g/dL. It is important that the nurse assess the patient, not just the number. Some patients do not tolerate hemoglobin levels ≤ 9.0 g/dL, and if patients are symptomatic, they should receive transfusions sooner.

28. List symptoms that indicate a patient needs a packed red blood cell transfusion.
Tachycardia
Pale skin color (including lips and nailbeds)
Fatigue
Irritability
Dizziness
Headaches
Shortness of breath

29. What is a normal platelet count?
$150–450 \times 10^9$/L. Patients who receive cancer therapy are frequently **thrombocytopenic** (low platelet count) and rarely have a platelet count this high.

30. When is a platelet transfusion indicated?
Whether or not a patient requires a transfusion may vary depending on the patient, his or her diagnosis, and whether or not a procedure is being done. In general, patients receive a transfusion if the platelet count is $< 10–20 \times 10^9$/L. For platelet counts $> 20 \times 10^9$/L but $< 50 \times 10^9$/L, a patient may receive a transfusion only if there is evidence of bleeding. Children with brain tumors receive a transfusion when the platelet count is $< 50 \times 10^9$/L because of the increased risk for intracranial bleeding with platelet counts less than that. If an invasive procedure (i.e., lumbar puncture or bone marrow aspirate) or other surgery is scheduled, a transfusion may be given to prevent bleeding, even if the count does not appear to be low.

31. If the risk of significant bleeding occurs with platelet counts $< 50 \times 10^9$/L, why not transfuse the patient for any value less than that?
Patients who can tolerate lower platelet counts are permitted to do so because frequent transfusions may lead to antibody development. The more transfusions a patient receives, the greater chance that he or she will develop antibodies that inhibit platelets. The more platelet transfusions given, the better chance antibodies will develop, and the less effective each transfusion may be. If a patient in the early stage of therapy receives a transfusion, the platelet count may increase from 10×10^9/L pretransfusion to 80×10^9/L post-transfusion. Over the course of a year or more of intensive therapy and frequent transfusions, the platelets may rise only from 10×10^9/L to 20×10^9/L with each transfusion, and it becomes increasingly difficult to manage platelet requirements and bleeding.

32. List interventions to reduce the risk of bleeding in a thrombocytopenic patient.
- Assess daily for **petechiae** (fine red freckle spots), increased or abnormal bruising, nosebleeds, and bleeding gums.
- Use a soft toothbrush or toothette; avoid flossing.
- Avoid administration of intramuscular or subcutaneous injections. If absolutely necessary, apply firm pressure to injection site for at least 5–10 minutes to avoid excessive bleeding and hematoma formation.
- Assess carefully for covert signs of bleeding: dipstick urine for heme and guaiac stools.
- Advise patients to restrict physical activity: no rough play, no climbing or jumping (to avoid falls), and no sharp toys.

33. List nursing tasks to be done before administering any chemotherapeutic agent.
   1. Verify informed consent, and provide patient education regarding the details of the regimen and anticipated side effects. Provide written information when available.

2. Review laboratory data (complete blood count, electrolytes, uric acid).

3. Double-check all calculations: check height, weight, and body surface area, and recalculate dosage of medications with another nurse.

4. Verify order for name, dosage, route, rate, and frequency.

5. Have emergency medications and equipment available.

34. Discuss the role of radiation therapy in the treatment of pediatric cancers.

The goal of **radiation therapy** is to deliver a therapeutic dose of ionizing radiation to eliminate malignant cells in the CNS and other sanctuary sites, while minimizing the injury to surrounding healthy tissues. Because chemotherapy alone may not treat these sites, radiation is given as an **adjuvant therapy**. Ionizing radiation has a direct effect on the target cells by affecting the DNA's ability to replicate. Loss of the cells' reproductive capacity is considered to be the most biologically significant end point of radiation.

35. How is radiation delivered?

Total-body irradiation is commonly used in stem cell transplant to eradicate cancer cells throughout the body and to enhance engraftment of stem cells by suppressing the body's immune response. It is given in fractionated doses at least 6 hours apart over 3–4 days. Each treatment lasts about 15 minutes and requires the patient to remain absolutely still for the duration of the therapy. Patients often may require sedation. Important aspects of treatment delivery include administration of a uniform dose of radiation to the entire body, provision of adequate lung shielding, and attention to the radiation time-dose interval.

Local control irradiation may be given to patients with solid tumors or lymphoma or patients with leukemia who are at high risk for developing CNS disease. It usually is given daily over 10–15 minutes and, depending on the areas to be irradiated, may take 1 week to several months to complete.

Total lymphoid irradiation focuses on radiating all the lymphoid-producing cells in the body. Total lymphoid irradiation has the potential benefit of contributing the desirable T-cell immunosuppressive effects with potentially less host toxicity than is experienced with total-body irradiation. It is administered similarly to local control radiation.

36. Describe the major acute toxicities of radiation therapy and how they can be minimized.

Skin desquamation. Initially, skin does not appear to be affected by radiation. After about 2–4 weeks, the skin may become darkened, dry, rough, erythematous, and desquamated. The patient should be instructed to use a thin moisturizing cream twice a day during the therapy. The patient should avoid creams that contain alcohol or anything that may be irritating and try to avoid scratching because of the risk of infection. When radiation is complete, the skin usually heals over several weeks.

Severe mucositis. This can be extremely painful and difficult to manage. A basic mouth care regimen of saline and baking soda mouth rinses every 2–3 hours is advised. If the pain increases, a combination of diphenhydramine, viscous lidocaine, and aluminum hydroxide with magnesium hydroxide (Mylanta or Maalox) may be used to numb the area and provide temporary pain relief. Patients commonly require narcotic analgesics during times of severe mucositis.

Nausea and vomiting. This commonly occurs with total-body irradiation. Patients can be premedicated for their therapy with an antiemetic of choice, which often provides significant relief.

37. List delayed toxicities of radiation therapy.

Growth abnormalities
Endocrine disorders
Cataracts
Secondary malignancies

38. List the major complications of stem cell transplant.
- Mouth sores, vomiting, diarrhea, and loss of appetite
- Bleeding resulting from insufficient platelet production
- Darkening or blistering of the skin
- Infection—because high doses of chemotherapy and radiotherapy are given during transplant, patients have prolonged periods of **neutropenia** and **immunosuppression**. This puts them at a significantly increased risk for infection.
- Liver complications—high-dose chemotherapy and radiation to the abdomen can cause liver damage.
- Lung and heart problems—the lungs and heart may be weakened by high-dose chemotherapy, and the lungs may be congested because of the large amounts of fluid that must be given.
- Graft-versus-host disease (GVHD)
- Late effects—sterility, growth retardation, endocrine dysfunction, and secondary malignancies

39. What is GVHD?
A complication of allogeneic blood or marrow transplantation. GVHD can occur whenever blood or bone marrow from one person is transfused into the bloodstream of another person whose immune system is suppressed as a result of medications or genetic defects. When the stem cells from the donor are infused into the patient, some of the donor's immune cells also are infused. GVHD occurs when some of the immune cells from the donor begin to react against certain tissues in the body. Before the stem cell infusion, patients start medications that help prevent GVHD. These medications may continue for 1 year after the transplant.

40. Summarize the different types of stem cell transplant and their indications.

TYPE OF TRANSPLANT	STEM CELL SOURCE	HOW IT WORKS	INDICATIONS
Autologous	Patient's own stem cells collected either by bone marrow harvest or by apheresis	Allows patients to receive higher doses of chemotherapy and/or radiotherapy that in normal circumstances would be too toxic for the marrow to recover	Malignant disease: Lymphomas Neuroblastoma Relapsed Wilms' tumor CNS tumors Other solid tumors (Ewing's sarcoma, rhabdomyosarcoma, desmoplastic small round cell tumor
Allogeneic	Stem cells from another human being, other than an identical twin May include Matched or mismatched family member Unrelated adult donors Umbilical cord blood (related or unrelated)	Has two primary aims: To eliminate remaining cancer cells in the body To replace the patient's bone marrow with donor cells that not only do not have cancer, but also will recognize any residual cancer cells as foreign and attack them to maintain long-term remission (graftversus-tumor effect)	Leukemias: ALL, acute myeloid leukemia, chronic myelogenous leukemia, JMML Lymphomas: Hodgkin's and non-Hodgkin's Nonmalignant diseases: Genetic disorders Hemoglobin disorders Bone marrow failure syndromes Metabolic and genetic disorders Immunologic disorders Autoimmune disorders Histiocytosis

Continued on following page

TYPE OF TRANSPLANT	STEM CELL SOURCE	HOW IT WORKS	INDICATIONS
Syngeneic	Stem cells from an identical twin	Replaces the abnormal functioning stem cells with new healthy cells	Has been used in aplastic anemia and other selected malignant and nonmalignant diseases
		There is little risk for GVHD with this type of transplant, which may be harmful or beneficial depending on diagnosis	Not used for diseases in which graft-versus-tumor effect is desired because there is rarely GVHD with these these transplants
			May be given without any chemotherapy or radiotherapy before cell infusion

ALL = acute lymphoblastic leukemia, JMML = juvenile myelomonocytic leukemia.

BIBLIOGRAPHY

1. Guidelines for preventing opportunistic infections among hematopoietic stem cell transplant recipients: Recommendations of the CDC, IDSA, and ASBMT, October 20, 2000. MMWR Morb Mortal Wkly Rep 49(RR10):1–128, 2000.
2. Hudak C, Gallo B, Benz J (eds): Critical Care Nursing: A Holistic Approach, 5th ed. Philadelphia, J.B. Lippincott, 1990.
3. Pizzo PA, Poplack DG (eds): Principles and Practice of Pediatric Oncology, 3rd ed. Philadelphia, Lippincott-Raven, 1997.
4. Thomas ED, Blume K, Forman S (eds): Hematopoietic Cell Transplantation, 2nd ed. Malden, MA, Blackwell Science, 1999.

14. MENTAL HEALTH CONDITIONS OF THE CHILD

Bruce K. Wilson, PhD

1. What causes mental disorders in children?

Although a definite cause of a mental disorder can be identified in some cases, in general the causes of mental disorders and factors involved remain unknown. Even when a specific cause can be identified, such as a period of **anoxia**, mitigating factors remain elusive.

2. How do cultural factors affect a child's mental health?

Culture largely determines what is viewed as **normal behavior** and **abnormal behavior**. Culture dictates how deviations from normal behavior are viewed and how the behaviors are classified and treated. In Canada and the United States, mental illness generally is viewed as different than physical illness. In the United States, insurance policies tend to pay differently for physical and mental health disruptions, and in general mental health conditions are viewed with a greater degree of shame and embarrassment. Children with gastroenteritis are not told to "get over it," but instead are taken to a practitioner for treatment. Children with depression or anxiety frequently are told to cure themselves.

Within subcultures, various views of mental health and illness may differ. Many parents prefer that a physiologic cause for the disturbance be identified. Others would prefer that their child be labeled as "emotionally ill" rather than "mentally ill." Health care providers need to be sensitive to the family's views.

Children learn from their culture what can be revealed and what must be hidden. Children in some cultures view talking to dead relatives as natural, whereas some health care practitioners might see this as psychotic. A child in one culture may be taught that it is appropriate to cry, whereas a different culture may teach the child that crying is bad. It is important that health care practitioners are aware of the cultural background of the child.

3. Discuss potential biologic factors in mental disorders.

A wide variety of prenatal, intranatal, and postnatal factors affect the child's mental health. With the massive amount of genetic research now being conducted, many underlying **genetic** factors are starting to surface.

Other factors with a biologic effect include various **toxins** in the environment. **Heavy metals**, such as lead, mercury, and arsenic, affect a child much more than an adult because the child is still developing. **Chemicals** placed on floors may not harm adults but may damage young children severely because children play on the floors.

Pain studies show that infants experiencing severe pain shortly after birth react more to pain experienced later. This indicates that there are **physiologic changes** in children based on the sensations they experience.

4. What is the fragile X syndrome?

In 1991, a genetic defect in the **X chromosome** was shown to cause a variety of mental defects, ranging from conduct disorders to retardation to autism. Individuals with this disorder also tend to have hyperextensible joints, long faces, and large ears. A defective *FMR1* gene on the long arm of the chromosome causes the syndrome. The genetic permutation causes a decrease in the amount of the fragile X protein. It is estimated that this syndrome affects approximately 1 of 2000 males and 1 of 4000 females. Large-scale studies are still needed, but this may be one of the most common genetic defects in humans. Females usually are affected less than males because they have a second X chromosome. In 1999, a study showed that two monozygotic (identical) twins had differences in the degree of the genetic disturbance, and the twin with the greater disturbance had increased mental defects. Some factor slightly different within the uterus caused these two individuals to develop different chromosomal conditions and different mental disorders; this indicates there is a potential for modifying the intrauterine environment to improve mental outcomes.

5. Describe how children grieve their losses.

Children grieve based on their developmental level, past experience with losses, and the amount of other stressors in their life. **Toddlers** start playing peek-a-boo when they learn that objects exist even when they are not seen. Through the **preschool** years, children tend to have unique ideas about what it means to be dead and what it means to be alive. They may think they caused the death by their thoughts or that the dead person will "wake up" if they behave correctly. They may regress in some behaviors. At this age, children may grieve the loss of items as much as the death of a family member. A preschooler moving to a different city may grieve the loss of his or her home, neighborhood, and friends.

Starting about the time children start **school**, they realize that death is permanent and begin to realize that all people die. They may be confused about some of the rituals of death and sometimes frightened by the rituals. When facing the death of one close individual, they may fear their own death or the death of others.

Children are sensitive to the feelings of their adult caretakers and frequently feel that they caused or are responsible for the adult's feelings. Some adults try to hide their feelings, and this tends to confuse the child further. In the case of a divorce, children may believe they caused the divorce and be grieving the loss of the intact family and the changes in their life.

When a caregiver or close friend dies, a child may feel **abandonment**. The child feels the person purposely left them alone. The child may also feel abandoned by other adults who are caught up in their own grief. If a sibling dies, the child may grieve the loss of the sibling and grieve the loss of the grieving parents.

Children frequently express their grief **behaviorally**. They may act afraid or unruly. Some children become withdrawn and interact minimally with their environment.

6. What is an adjustment disorder?

A severe reaction to a loss that begins within 3 months of the loss and shows no signs of dwindling. Generally, it is a sign that the child is having problems working through grief, and frequently well-meaning adults may compound the problem. Children grieve their losses. If they are "required" to hide the process, they may express the loss in other ways or be unable to resolve the loss. The more the child is told to ignore the loss and concentrate on other things, the more the child can become focused on the loss.

7. List symptoms of adjustment disorders.
   • An excessive, lengthy focusing only on the loss
   • A sharp decrease in school performance or refusal to attend school
   • A lack of interest in all friends or play activities
   • An inability to return to normal activities after several weeks
   • Extended anger at parents or other surviving family members
   • Frequently expressing a desire to join the dead person

8. How can nurses help children work through the grieving process?

Nurses can help children by giving them permission to express their feelings and to ask questions. When a child asks questions that enter the area of **religious belief**, the nurse can help best by turning the question around and asking what the child has heard about death in the child's religion or asking if the child would like to ask one of his or her religious leaders. The nurse does not have to pretend to be an expert in death. Children normally are most concerned about their own safety and who will take care of them.

Children also need a time to be **distracted from grieving**. Grieving is hard work, and the child may need permission to forget about the loss and concentrate on a game or reading a book. The key is to ask the child what he or she wants to do and to make suggestions without pressure. If a parent is also grieving, the child needs to be told that this is a temporary situation. The parent has not forgotten about the child but is busy right now. Most children understand that parents can be busy with other things, yet still care about them.

9. How should nurses instruct parents to care for themselves?

Adults caring for children need to realize when they need a break or even other assistance. Adults should remember to get outside help for themselves and the children. Parents need to be helped to understand how children are grieving. Sometimes parents mistakenly believe that if they pretend nothing happened, children will recover faster. If this happens, children may wonder if parents would miss them if they died, or children may hide their feelings to please their parents. Children should not be led to believe that their job is to replace the missing person. Telling a child, "You have to be the man [or woman] of the house now," puts a tremendous burden on the child.

10. What can nurses do to help children in times of disaster?

For children, a major **disaster** is anything that disrupts their lives and their feeling of safety. For children, the major question is always, **"Am I safe?"** Modern media frequently provide constant coverage of disasters, and adults tend to focus on the events as a way of coping. These images are extremely frightening to children. One of the first things to do to help children is to decrease the intensity of the stimuli they are receiving. If it is necessary to receive possible evacuation data, listening to the radio is less traumatizing than watching the images on the television.

Children need to be reminded of all the things done to keep them safe. If the disaster is far away, children need to be reminded that it is occurring in another place. It is reassuring to children to review plans such as a fire evacuation plan and how they fit into the plan. Sometimes, helping children to plan how they will save one of their favorite items will comfort them.

Children need to be permitted to express their feelings and have the feelings accepted. After the World Trade Center destruction in 2001, one group of fourth graders was most upset that Disney World was closed. Their teacher comforted them by telling them that this was only temporary. Another helpful activity is to permit children to help others in some way. It may be to donate a toy or part of the child's allowance, send a card, or pick out old clothes to donate. Children, similar to adults, feel less helpless if they are permitted actively to help.

11. What can the nurse expect of the behavior of a child after a disaster?

- As with any loss, children may **regress** to earlier behaviors and become unusually clingy.
- Children at home may need to be reassured frequently of the parent's presence.
- Schools and hospitals need to provide children with a way to contact their parents for reassurance.
- Hospitalized children may need to be assured of the nurse's presence.

Knowing that they can contact adult caregivers if necessary can relieve much of the anxiety for children.

12. Why do nurses need to pay attention to psychological labels?

Psychological and psychiatric labels are important to staff nurses in the same way other medical diagnoses are important to nurses. If a patient had a surgical procedure the previous day, the competent nurse takes steps to minimize and treat the expected pain. If a patient has a mental condition, the nurse also takes steps to make the patient more comfortable.

13. How does the nurse make a patient with a mental condition more comfortable?

Making the patient **comfortable** does not mean always meeting all the patient's demands, but rather creating a **safe environment** with minimal distress and discomfort. Sometimes, by giving in to a controlling child, the child becomes more out of control trying to find the limits.

14. Does the label (diagnosis) help or hurt the child with a mental disorder?

Different children and their families react differently to having a mental health diagnosis. Frequently, for families in which the disorder has caused a large amount of disruption, having a diagnosis provides a sense of relief: They finally are told that it is a real problem and there are potential treatments. On the other hand, some families deny the diagnosis and believe that the diagnosis labels the child as a problem child. For professionals, the label provides a method of communicating the nature of the problem.

15. Define learning disabilities.

A child with a learning disability may have problems getting information, processing the information, or responding to the information. For a child to hear a word and write the word on paper, the child first must have relatively normal hearing, then transmit the message to the neurons where the sound is interpreted, then transmit that message to the area where the message is understood, then transmit the message to the area that controls spelling, then convey the message to the motor area, then convey the message to the hand that performs the writing, and while learning the skill simultaneously confirm the action with sight and touch. Different children have abilities and disabilities in learning, just as children have differing skills on the athletic field. In these cases, the diagnosis does not identify the actual problem, but rather the **lack of ability** that is the result of the problem.

16. How are learning disabilities treated?

An important part of treatment is to decrease the impact of the deficit and to assist children in optimizing their abilities. If a child has a visual problem and needs glasses, the child is fitted with the appropriate corrective lenses and taught how to deal with the actions of others in response to the glasses. If a child has a problem with spelling or mathematical ability the same approach should be taken.

17. What are expressive disabilities?

Disabilities involved with **impaired communication**. These range from slow or faulty language development to stuttering and Tourette's syndrome. **Tourette's syndrome** is characterized by motor and vocal tics. Some individuals with Tourette's syndrome are unable to control voicing socially unacceptable words or phrases. These vocalizations are not deliberate and are not under the individual's control. The best response to Tourette's syndrome and other expressive disorders is to relax to permit the individual to communicate without interruption.

18. Why do children who are learning two or more languages seem to have an expressive disorder?

These children actually are trying to sort out different concepts and dual words for the same object. Studies indicate that they eventually develop greater verbal ability.

19. Define mental retardation.

Intelligence is measured on an **intelligence quotient (IQ)** scale based on a score of 100 being average. Mentally retarded individuals have significantly below-normal levels of intelligence and a decreased learning ability. Individuals with other deficits may be incorrectly labeled as retarded because of the difficulty in testing.

20. Classify the levels of mental retardation.

IQ	LEVEL OF MENTAL RETARDATION	CHARACTERISTICS
50–70	Mild	Most mentally retarded are in this category Can achieve skills of a 6th-grader Can achieve self-sufficiency with some support
35–50	Moderate	Can achieve skills of a 2nd grader Can participate in some work and social activities with supervision
20–35	Severe	Can perform some self-care activities with supervision
< 20	Profound	< 2% of mentally retarded persons Need total care

21. What are pervasive developmental disorders?

Disorders that are characterized by major disturbances in thinking, learning, communicating, and socialization. The most striking aspect of these diseases is the **lack of normal social interactions** or the extremely abnormal social interactions.

22. List pervasive developmental disorders.

Autism
Rett's syndrome
Childhood disintegration disorder
Childhood schizophrenia
Asperger's disorder

23. Describe autism.

Autism, the most commonly known pervasive developmental disorder, is characterized by:
- Onset before the age of 3
- Failure to develop normal interactions with the environment
- Lack of appropriate verbal and nonverbal communications
- Lack of awareness of self and others
- Engagement in acts that are destructive to themselves and others

24. What are the characteristics of Rett's syndrome?

Children with this permanent condition usually develop normally until about age 4 years, when the following signs and symptoms become evident:
- Loss of acquired social skills
- Normal head circumference at birth that slows to below normal (slowing may begin as early as age 5 months)
- Loss of physical abilities

25. Describe childhood disintegrative disorder.

Children with childhood disintegrative disorder develop normally for the first 2 years. Between the ages of 2 and 10 years, the child starts to lose skills and presents behaviors similar to the child with autism. The decline in abilities may stop at any level, and the child may show slight improvement.

26. Describe Asperger's disorder.

Asperger's disorder is similar to autism except that children with Asperger's do not have the impaired language skills. The main characteristic is severely disturbed social interactions. These children do not have impaired cognitive ability and may become focused on learning about a specific area. Some of these children may be misdiagnosed with behavioral disorders or with attention-deficit disorder.

27. Describe childhood schizophrenia.

Similar to adult-onset schizophrenia, childhood schizophrenia is characterized by bizarre delusions and hallucinations, occurring after normal development. These delusions and hallucinations last longer than 1 month and are not related to the typical **magical thinking** that characterizes the preschool years.

28. What special care does the pediatric nurse need to give to a child with a pervasive developmental disorder?

The key aspect of care is **consistency**. The world is a scary place for these children, and any change in routine or personnel results in an increase in symptoms and aggressive behavior. Whenever possible, the same individual should provide all the care.

29. Do children develop depression?

Children suffer from **depression** and **bipolar depression**. Depression is not associated with a specific event, although it may be precipitated by one event or a series of events. Children with depression may become withdrawn, engage in aggressive acting out, or show an inability to concentrate. Current research indicates that one of the factors in depression is an imbalance in **neurotransmitters**.

30. Do children commit suicide?

Yes. Suicide is a leading cause of death among **adolescents**. It is the sixth leading cause of death in children between 5 and 14 years old and the third leading cause of death in individuals between ages 15 and 24. **Preschool children** may commit suicide in an effort to join a loved one who died, in an effort to see God, or in the belief that they will regain life like a cartoon character. **Older children** commit suicide because they are unable to see any other way out of their pain. Boys are substantially more successful in suicide attempts than girls.

31. How should anxiety (fear and phobias) in childhood be handled?

Children normally have many fears. The paradox is that many times they are not afraid of situations that are dangerous and may be terrified by things that are not dangerous.

Preschool children typically are terrified of "monsters" in the dark. Using a night-light or giving the child a flashlight may be all the intervention needed.

A **sudden onset** of fearful behavior may indicate the child recently has experienced a terrifying event related to the fear. It may have been a comment by an adult or something viewed on television or in a movie.

- If the response to the fear is not a great disruption to a child's life, it is usually best to provide a sense of security and avoid the stimulus.
- If the stimulus or feared object cannot be avoided, the child can be supported in becoming more comfortable with the object.

Children tend to pick up fears of their parents and be calmed by a lack of fear in their parents.

32. What about school phobia, or when the child refuses to go to school?

This is an example of a fear that cannot be avoided. The longer the child does not go to school, the greater the fear grows. Most experts agree that the child should be forced to attend school. Caregivers should try to determine if there is a specific thing the child is afraid of, such as a bully or fear of wetting his or her pants. These specific fears can be addressed.

33. Differentiate between normal behavioral problems and severe behavioral problems.

All children tell lies, misbehave, and are not respectful of the rights of others at times. Normally, corrective action by parents and teachers resolve the problem, and there are minimal recurrences. For some children, owing to their nature, physiology, or the lack of effective correction in the past, the behavior becomes substantially worse, and the usual corrective actions are ineffective.

34. What is a conduct disorder?

A child with a conduct disorder repeatedly violates rules and the rights of others over time. These behaviors include acts of **physical cruelty** to people or animals and may involve **setting fires**. The child must be capable intellectually and developmentally of recognizing these violations. The behavior disrupts the social, occupational, or academic functioning of the child. Children with this disorder need to be monitored closely to minimize the harm they do and prevent the secondary gains from their activity. In treatment, these children frequently acknowledge feelings of powerlessness and fear after they have dropped their initial bluff of bravado.

35. What is oppositional defiant disorder?

Children with this disorder direct their hostility and disability against individuals in authority. They tend to see rules as unreasonable and their actions of rule violations as appropriate. With health care practitioners or teachers, the behavior may not be visible. The severity of this disorder tends to increase over time if not treated successfully.

36. Discuss attention-deficit disorder.

This disorder is diagnosed when a child has difficulty maintaining attention for an appropriate time for the child's developmental level. This may be recognized more in boys because they mature neurologically about 2 years later than girls. This disorder is recognized most commonly in children who are hyperactive in school settings. Many mothers tell of years of trying to keep up with the child. The child may be literally bouncing off the walls, running from task to task, and surviving on a few hours of sleep. Paradoxically, **stimulant medications** help many of these children focus their attention. Decreasing the amount of stimulation also helps the child concentrate.

37. How should the family first seek help for a mental health or behavioral problem?

The easiest and most effective place to start the evaluation process is with a complete **physical examination**, including complete **endocrine studies**. Many behavioral or mental problems are resolved after an underlying problem, such as hypoglycemia or a thyroid disorder, is discovered and treated. If a child is not responding after 6 months of medical therapy, a complete battery of **psychological tests** should be performed. Generally, school districts are required to provide the psychological testing.

38. State a problem for families when seeking treatment for a mental health or behavior problem.

Because the symptoms are frequently similar, a child might be treated for the wrong syndrome, leading to frustration and guilt.

39. How does play therapy help children?

Children's natural world is one of play. Through their use of **toys**, children frequently show their understanding of how they feel, how they view the world, and how they view their conflicts. With professional assistance, children often can work through conflicts in play activities.

40. How is art therapy used?

Art therapy is similar to play therapy. By using various media, the child expresses feelings and views and begins working out conflicts. Care must be taken always to permit the child to discuss the creation rather than the adult ascribing the meaning. Asking open-ended questions, such as "tell me about this picture," is much better than asking the child if the picture has a specific meaning. A child may draw himself or herself as separated from the family because at that moment he or she is alone and the other family members are elsewhere.

41. What are the characteristics of behavioral therapy?
- Behavioral therapy provides **consistent** responses to the child's actions.
- It is important that the hospitalized child receive the same responses.
- Behavioral therapy works only if applied all the time.
- **Rewards** are established for appropriate behavior, and **consequences** are established for undesirable behaviors.
- Behavioral therapy addresses the behavior, not the reasons behind the behavior.

42. Why is family therapy important if the problem is with the child?
The child's behavior affects the family, and the family's behavior affects the child. The child may be behaving inappropriately to distract attention from other conflicts within the family, and frequently if the "problem" child changes his or her behavior, another family member may start to exhibit inappropriate behavior.

43. What is the pediatric nurse's role in identifying a child with a mental condition?
The pediatric nurse is in the unique position of seeing numerous children in differing situations over a length of time. Physicians may see the child only for brief periods, and parents may see only their own child. The nurse needs to identify behavior outside the normal and make a referral when necessary.

Examples. In one case, the nurse insisted a physician consider that a particular child was unusually irritable. A spinal tap revealed the child had bacterial meningitis. Early treatment prevented neurologic damage. In another case, an external evaluator decided that a child had a severe developmental delay on the Denver Developmental Screening Test. The evaluator stated that the child did not know the words for horse or dog in either language that was common in the area. The nurse had just been looking at a picture book with the child and pointed out that the child called a horse a "pony" and a dog a "puppy." The words were a reflection of the child's background, not underlying disability.

CONTROVERSIES

44. What role do medications play in childhood mental disorders?
A variety of medications are used in treating childhood mental disorders. The long-term safety of many of these has not been shown. At times, the child initially responds to one medication, but the response decreases with time. At this time, most medications are used only to control the child's symptoms and not to treat the underlying disorder.

45. Discuss the role of complementary therapies in childhood mental conditions.
Some groups have advocated **nutritional therapy** and **environmental therapies**, such as removing allergens. Many parents report improvement resulting from these activities, although research has not shown consistent results except in limited cases, such as phenylketonuria. Generally, if the therapy is not harmful to the child, families should not be discouraged from trying complementary therapies.

BIBLIOGRAPHY
1. American Psychiatric Association: Diagnostic and Statistical Manual of Mental Disorders, 4th ed., text revision. Washington, DC, American Psychiatric Association, 2001.
2. Copel LC: Nurses Clinical Guide to Psychiatric Mental Health Care, 2nd ed. Springhouse, PA, Springhouse Corporation, 2000.
3. Helderman-van den Enden ATJM, Maaswinkel-Mooij PD, Hoogendoorn E, et al: Monozygotic twin brothers with the fragile X syndrome: Different CGG repeats and different mental capacities. J Med Genet 36:53–57, 1999.
4. Seligman ME, Walker EF, Rosenhan DL: Abnormal Psychology, 4th ed. New York, W.W. Norton, 2001.

15. INFECTIOUS DISEASES OF CHILDHOOD

Barbara Hoyer Schaffner, PhD, RN, CPNP

1. Name the most common bacterial infection in children.
Acute otitis media.

2. What is the incidence of acute otitis media?
Otitis media occurs in 70% of children younger than 3 years, with a greater occurrence in boys than girls. The incidence has increased 2.5-fold in 25 years.

3. List risk factors for the development of acute otitis media.
- Very low birth weight
- Preterm birth
- Male gender
- Crowding (specifically, attending day care)
- Exposure to parental smoking
- Pacifier use past 6 months of age
- Sibling history of recurrent otitis media

4. What factors help protect against acute otitis media?
Female gender
Breast-feeding
Infant sleeping in the supine position

5. What factors are not associated with acute otitis media?
Maternal use of prenatal drugs, alcohol, or medication
Prenatal diet
Maternal illness during the third trimester

6. How is acute otitis media treated?
Antibiotics, beginning with the **penicillins**.

7. Which other antibiotics can be used in addition to penicillin?
Second-generation cephalosporins
Third-generation cephalosporins
Macrolides
Fluoroquinolones

8. What age group has been newly identified as being at increased risk for meningococcal meningitis?
Meningitis from *Neisseria meningitidis* has emerged as one of the next bacteria causing an increase in the number of meningitis cases, affecting especially **adolescents** and **young adults**. The highest rate of infection has been found in freshmen students living in dormitory settings.

9. What about meningitis resulting from *Haemophilus influenzae* type b?
Meningitis from *H. influenzae* type b has been virtually eliminated as a result of effective immunizations of infants and young children with the **HIB vaccine**.

10. List risk factors for meningococcal infection.
- Contact with someone known to have the disease
- Crowding

- On-campus residence
- Cigarette smoking
- Campus-area bar patronage, especially more than one bar

11. Describe the signs and symptoms of meningococcal infection.

Early meningococcal infection is difficult to distinguish from benign viral infections. Many complain initially of **flulike symptoms**, with fever, headache, malaise, congestion, nausea, vomiting, and anorexia. The characteristic features of meningococcal disease appear **later** on and include rash, altered mental status, and meningism.

12. What infectious disease has been found in public swimming pools?

Since the summer of 2000, outbreaks of *Cryptosporidium* have been documented in public swimming pools, causing widespread **infectious diarrhea**.

13. What are the symptoms of cryptosporidiosis?

Diarrhea
Abdominal cramps
Anorexia
Nausea and vomiting

14. How is cryptosporidiosis spread in swimming pools?

Spread is thought to be by fecal accident of one swimmer, who then exposes the other swimmers.

15. What are the Centers for Disease Control and Prevention (CDC) recommendations for pool design and management to prevent further incidents of *Cryptosporidium* infection?

- No swimming should be allowed by persons with diarrhea while ill and for 2 weeks after diarrhea has resolved.
- Immunocompromised individuals should not swim at all during known outbreaks.
- Swimmers should be careful not to swallow pool water.
- Good hygiene should be practiced before swimming, when using the restroom, and after changing diapers.
- Ensure frequent bathroom breaks for children when at the pool.

16. What can be the problem when children get red eyes?

Conjunctivitis.

17. What are the presenting symptoms of conjunctivitis?

Watery, burning eyes that are swollen and edematous.

18. Differentiate among the three types of conjunctivitis.

1. **Bacterial** conjunctivitis has a purulent discharge. It is more common in children younger than 6 years old.
2. **Viral** conjunctivitis has a watery discharge. It is more common in children older than age 6.
3. **Allergic** conjunctivitis has a stringy discharge.

19. What is the treatment for bacterial conjunctivitis?

Prescription eye antibiotic ointment or drops.

20. What are styes?

Acute inflammations along the lid margins; these can be treated with warm compresses in the home setting.

21. How common is tinea capitis?

Tinea capitis is an increasing public health concern in the United States. It has been found to be increasing in certain populations, specifically among **African Americans**. It is found most often in urban areas, particularly **inner cities**. Children **3–7 years old** are most likely to have tinea capitis.

22. How does tinea capitis present?

1. The **noninflammatory** type is characterized by the breaking of the hair just above the level of the scalp, leaving the characteristic black-dot ringworm appearance.

2. The **inflammatory** type is characterized by papules, pustules, and crusting in the hair that resembles a seborrheic dermatitis.

23. What is the suggested treatment for tinea capitis?

Because of the involvement of the hair follicles, tinea capitis is treated with oral antifungal medication. First-line therapy is **griseofulvin**, 15–25 mg/kg/day, taken until scaling has ceased and hair is growing in the area, which can be 8–12 weeks. To increase absorption, griseofulvin should be taken with fatty foods.

24. Which infectious rash is associated with wrestling?

Tinea corporis is a red scaly rash that is usually seen on the lower arms and legs, whereas **tinea gladiatorum** is usually seen on the neck, head, and shoulders. An increase in the number of children participating in wrestling has been associated with the increase in tinea. If one member of the wrestling team is diagnosed with tinea, teammates should be checked periodically, and team mats and headgear should be treated with a fungicide. A child with tinea should be placed on antifungal medication and excluded from competition if the lesions are exposed.

25. What is fifth disease?

Erythema infectiosum, a mild childhood disease characterized by low-grade fever, malaise, and a sore throat, which is caused by **parvovirus B19** and spread by **respiratory secretions**. The incubation period is 6–16 days. The classic sign is the **facial rash** that resembles a **slapped cheek** appearance over the malar areas of the face, which appears 1–4 days after the initial symptoms. The facial rash is followed by a diffuse macular or maculopapular rash on the extremities and trunk. The rash may last 10 days and is pruritic in half of the cases reported. The child is no longer infectious when the rash appears. Fifth disease can be dangerous to the unborn fetus, causing **hydrops fetalis** and **fetal death**, especially if the pregnant mother is infected before the 20th week of gestation.

26. What is sixth disease?

Roseola infantum, more commonly known simply as roseola, is a common acute illness of young children (usually < 2 years old), which presents with a sudden onset of **fever** that lasts 3–5 days. Roseola is caused by a variety of **viral agents**. The fever ends as quickly as it began. At the end of the fever, a discrete erythematous, macular rash appears primarily on the trunk. The rash blanches easily with pressure, lasts 24–48 hours, and is not associated with pruritus.

27. What are coxsackieviruses?

Group A coxsackieviruses are responsible for causing common mild viral illnesses in children, including **herpangina** and **hand-foot-and-mouth disease.**

28. Describe herpangina.

Herpangina is a self-limiting illness characterized by fever and painful vesicles and ulcers on the soft palate and tonsillar pillars. The illness can last 4–5 days. Treatment is symptomatic with **antipyretics** for fever and **topical medications** on painful oral lesions.

29. Describe hand-foot-and-mouth disease.

Hand-foot-and-mouth disease often is seen in **epidemics** in children younger than 4 years old. Vesicles appear in the mouth and on the palms of the hands and soles of the feet. The child appears mildly ill with malaise and a decrease in appetite. Treatment is symptomatic based on the specific discomfort of the child.

30. What is mononucleosis?

An illness caused by **Epstein-Barr virus**. The incubation period is thought to be 14–50 days. Most cases of mononucleosis develop in age-specific categories, mostly adolescents and young adults.

31. How is mononucleosis spread?

Through close personal contact between humans.

32. Describe the symptoms of mononucleosis.

The classic symptoms initially include malaise, fever, anorexia, and excessive fatigue. Many patients also complain of a severe sore throat with a presentation of exudative pharyngitis and tonsillar enlargement on physical examination. Generalized **lymphadenopathy** and **hepatosplenomegaly** develop within the first weeks.

33. How is mononucleosis diagnosed?

Laboratory evaluation of the **Monospot test** for patients older than age 4 years or **antibodies to Epstein-Barr virus** in children younger than 4 years and older patients with clinical signs of mononucleosis and a negative Monospot test.

34. What is the treatment for mononucleosis?

Supportive with rest, fluids, and avoidance of contact sports while hepatosplenomegaly is present.

35. What is varicella?

The virus that results in **chickenpox** in children. Reactivation of the latent virus can cause **shingles** in older children and adults.

36. Describe chickenpox.

An illness spread by respiratory droplets that is highly contagious, with 85% of infected contacts contracting the illness. The incubation period for chickenpox is 7–21 days. Most infections are seen in school-age children. Chickenpox is most commonly a mild illness with **low-grade fever** and a **vesicular rash**. Children are contagious until all lesions have crusted.

37. How severe is varicella infection?

Although chickenpox is mild, secondary infections can occur that include secondary skin infections (with staphylococci) and idiopathic thrombocytopenic purpura. Purpura fulminans and meningoencephalitis are rare complications.

38. How can the chickenpox rash be differentiated from other rashes?

Usually with chickenpox there is a known exposure within the community. The chickenpox rash is identifiable by the staging of the vesicles from **macules to papules to vesicles**. In most children, the rash includes lesions in all three forms at the time of initial diagnosis. The rash usually starts on the scalp or trunk and may involve the mucous membranes and sclera. It is usually pruritic. The rash usually spreads for the first 3-5 days.

39. What is the treatment for chickenpox?

Supportive with **acetaminophen** for fever and discomfort.

40. Discuss scarlet fever.

Scarlet fever is caused by **group A beta-hemolytic streptococci**. Most children have been infected with streptococcal organisms in the pharynx or tonsils and present with a **sore throat**. The rash is thought to be a result of a hypersensitization to toxins produced by the streptococcal organism. Scarlet fever rash is typically erythematous with fine papules placed close together, giving a characteristic sandpaper feel to the skin. The rash usually begins on the face and trunk.

41. How is scarlet fever diagnosed?

Throat culture or rapid streptococcus test.

42. What is the treatment for scarlet fever?

Penicillin VK in appropriate doses.

43. Is scarlet fever the same as rheumatic fever?

No, although they are related. Rheumatic fever is a combination of symptoms that occur as a sequel to nontreated or undertreated group A beta-hemolytic streptococcal infection. Symptoms of rheumatic fever range from rash to more systemic signs of arthritic pain, chorea, neurologic disorders, and the potential for mitral valve heart damage. The importance of treating scarlet fever and all group A beta-hemolytic streptococcal infections needs to be stressed to avoid the development of rheumatic fever and other possible complications from these infections.

44. What are the symptoms of pertussis?

- Coryza
- Sneezing
- Low-grade fever
- Cough that progresses to a rapid short paroxysmal cough that at the end has an inspiratory crowing sound sometimes referred to as a whoop

45. How is pertussis treated?

Treatment is with **antimicrobial** therapy, but the best treatment continues to be **prevention** through up-to-date **immunization**.

46. Why is there an increase in the number of cases of pertussis diagnosed in children?

The exact reason for the increase in pertussis is not clear, but one thought is that there is an increase in the diagnosis of pertussis. A second explanation, especially in children ages 10–14 years, is a **waning immunity** that develops approximately 7–10 years after the child's last **DTP (DTaP) booster**. Pertussis is most dangerous to infants, with an increase in reported infant deaths resulting from pertussis.

CONTROVERSIES

47. Are antibiotics necessary for the treatment of acute otitis media?

Concern exists about the overuse of antibiotics because such overuse and abuse leads to the emergence of resistant bacterial strains. A new **wait-and-see approach** for 72 hours is being advocated instead of the immediate prescription of antibiotics in all children with acute otitis media. The wait-and-see approach has been found to show no significant difference in mean pain scores, episodes of distress, or absence from school in children 6 months to 10 years of age. The group of children treated with antibiotics was found to have a shorter duration of symptoms, 1 day on average, but also was found to have a 10% higher incidence of diarrhea.

48. Should all college students be immunized against meningococcal disease?

The American College Health Association, the Advisory Committee on Immunization Practices of the Centers for Disease Control, and the American Academy of Pediatrics recommend that college freshmen, particularly those living in a dormitory, and their parents be educated about meningococcal disease and the vaccine so that they may make a decision on the need for student immunization.

BIBLIOGRAPHY

1. Alcorn DM: Red eye: When to treat and when to refer. Infect Dis Child 2001.
2. Centers for Disease Control: Cryptosporidiosis outbreaks from swimming pools. MMWR Morb Mortal Wkly Rep 50:406–410, 2001.
3. Cohen BA: Tinea capitis: Overview of the problem. Contemp Pediatr 3(suppl):3–5, 2001.
4. Croce G: Dutch pertussis outbreak may have been caused by antigenic changes. Infect Dis Child 13:101, 2000.
5. Harrison LH: Meningococcal infections in adolescents and young adults. Contemp Pediatr 4(suppl):4–15, 2001.
6. Little P, Gould C, Williamson I: Pragmatic randomised controlled trial of two prescribing strategies for childhood acute otitis media. BMJ 322:336, 2001.
7. Niemela M, Pihakari O, Pokka T: Pacifier as a risk factor for acute otitis media: A randomized controlled trial of parental counseling. Pediatrics 106:483, 2000.
8. Rosenthal TM: Periodic topical shampoo may be best treatment for tinea versicolor. Infect Dis Child 14:27, 2001.
9. Schwartz MW: Pediatric Primary Care: A Problem-Oriented Approach, 3rd ed. St. Louis, Mosby, 1997.
10. Wong DL: Whaley and Wong's Nursing Care of Infants and Children, 6th ed. St. Louis, Mosby, 1999.

16. IMMUNIZATIONS IN CHILDHOOD

Patricia Ryan-Krause, MS, RN, MSN, APRN

1. Why are immunizations important?

Immunizations are one of the most effective components of disease prevention and health promotion available to health care providers. As a result of immunization, smallpox has been eradicated from the world, and polio has been eliminated from the Americas. It is crucial to continue to administer vaccines because many causative organisms continue to exist in different parts of the world.

2. Identify reliable sources of information about current immunization practices.

The **American Academy of Pediatrics' *Red Book*** is an important source of information about common and less common issues concerning immunization. The **Centers for Disease Control and Prevention** provides definitive information about immunization schedules and practices for children and adults. These sources should be consulted for all questions regarding immunization administration, side effects, and schedules.

3. List five important facts about safe vaccine administration.

1. **Safe injection sites** include the anterior lateral aspect of the thigh for infants and young children and the deltoid muscle for older children. The thigh is the best site for multiple injections in infants and toddlers because of the large muscle mass.

2. Many experts and many package inserts suggest that the **syringe be aspirated** to ensure the vaccine is not being administered intravenously.

3. The needle for **intramuscular injections** must be long enough to reach the muscle to avoid injecting into the subcutaneous tissue.

4. **Disposable needles and syringes** should be used. Needles should not be recapped but placed immediately after use in a safe, puncture-proof, labeled container.

5. **Minor bleeding** at the site of the injection is expected and generally is stopped with slight pressure at the site.

4. Describe appropriate immunization practice in a sick child.

Minor illnesses, such as upper respiratory infections or gastroenteritis or other illnesses with or without a low-grade fever, generally are not contraindications to vaccine administration with live virus vaccines.

Moderate or severe illness with or without fever is a reason to defer immunization with diphtheria and tetanus toxoid and acellular pertussis (DTaP) because a subsequent fever may be difficult to distinguish from an immunization reaction.

Every effort must be made to immunize children with delayed immunizations. **Immunization records** should be reviewed at all illness and well-child visits and updated whenever possible.

5. Identify some approaches to take with parents who hesitate or refuse immunizations for their children.

- Take the time to listen to parents' questions and concerns.
- Identify specific religious or cultural issues that may be affecting their decisions.
- Ask about specific safety concerns that they may have.
- Ask if they have known anyone to have a serious reaction to any immunizations.
- Do not cite lengthy medical literature about immune response.
- Discuss the dramatic decrease in infectious, vaccine-preventable illness.
- Do not be coercive and threaten not to take care of the child.
- Continue to remind parents about benefits of immunizations at each encounter.

6. **What are some of the major barriers to delivery of immunizations?**
   • Socioeconomic—cost of vaccines to patients and providers
   • Late start of vaccines
   • Lack of information and awareness
   • Missed opportunities, lack of tracking, lack of reminders, deferment for minor illness
   • Office practices—waiting time, inconvenient hours for patients

7. **Is it okay to administer multiple vaccines at the same time?**
   Studies have shown that the immune response when single or multiple doses are administered is the same. Additionally, to improve immunization rates, it is appropriate to administer multiple vaccines at the same visit. DTaP, inactivated polio vaccine (IPV), *Haemophilus influenzae* b conjugate (HIB), and pneumococcal vaccine (PVC) frequently are administered at the same visit. There is no decrease in efficacy and no increase in adverse effects.

8. **When a child is significantly delayed in receiving immunizations, is it necessary to wait a certain interval between the administration of different vaccines?**
   If the measles, mumps, and rubella (MMR) and varicella (Varivax) vaccines are not given simultaneously (usually at 12–15 months), there must be a 1-month interval between administration of the MMR and Varivax. This interval reduces the risk of interference of one vaccine with another. All other different vaccines may be given without regard to interval. For example, if a child is delayed with immunizations, he or she could receive DaPT, IPV, HIB, and PVC-7 at one visit, then receive the MMR, Varivax, and hepatitis B at another visit, even in the same week.

9. **When is it necessary to restart an immunization series?**
   This is necessary only if the interval between the vaccines was too short (i.e., < 1 month between DTaP, HIB, IPV, and pneumococcal conjugates). The interval is never too great between immunizations (i.e., a child immunized at birth with hepatitis B can receive the second immunization at his or her kindergarten entry physical examination).

10. **How many DTaP vaccines should a child receive?**
    DTaP vaccines generally are administered at 2, 4, 6, and 12–15 months of age in healthy children. A booster dose is needed between 4 and 6 years of age at the time of school entry. If a child's immunization schedule has been delayed for any reason and the child receives the fourth dose of DTaP after the fourth birthday, a fifth dose is not needed. If a child still needs to complete the series for lapsed immunization after the seventh birthday, tetanus-diphtheria (TD) is administered, not DTaP, because of the reduced risk of pertussis after age 7 years.

11. **When is the DTaP vaccine contraindicated?**
    • An undetermined progressive neurologic disease.
    • Allergy to any components of an immunization.
    • A moderate degree of illness with or without a fever because it may be difficult to determine if a fever is a reaction to the vaccine or part of the illness.

12. **Are febrile seizures a contraindication to the administration of MMR or to DTaP?**
    No. Personal or family history of previous febrile seizure activity is not a contraindication because the **acellular pertussis vaccine** has a much lower risk of fever and subsequent seizure activity. Despite the possibility of fever after receiving the **MMR**, the risks of **underimmunization** outweigh the risks of a febrile seizure in the 7- to 10-day postvaccination time period when a child might experience a high fever. The risks of fever are low with the use of acellular pertussis so that the **DTaP** be given even to children who have experienced a febrile seizure. Careful fever prophylaxis should be reviewed with the caregivers.

13. When is the first booster with TD recommended?

A decrease in protection has been noted 6–10 years after the booster doses given at school entry (age 4–6 years), so it currently is recommended that the first booster be administered at **11 or 12 years** of age instead of 14–16 years. Subsequent boosters should be given every 10 years unless a patient experiences a **dirty wound**, such as a **deep puncture wound**. In this case, a TD is recommended if it has been more than 5 years since the last TD booster.

14. What types of wounds are more likely to be contaminated by *Clostridium tetani*?

Any open wound may be a source of **tetanus**, but wounds contaminated by dirt, feces, soil, or saliva have a higher risk of tetanus contamination than other wounds. Crush injuries, avulsion injuries, frostbite, and other wounds that may contain devitalized tissue are at increased risk for contamination with tetanus.

15. When is it necessary for a patient to have tetanus prophylaxis?

When a patient incurs a wound as described in question 14 and has a documented history of at least three doses of tetanus toxoid with the last dose being > 5 years ago, a **tetanus toxoid booster** is needed. If a person incurs a minor wound and has had three tetanus doses in the past, a tetanus booster is not needed unless it has been > 10 years since the last dose of tetanus toxoid.

16. When is tetanus immunoglobulin indicated?

This additional vaccine is needed if a person incurs a serious wound as described in question 14 and has not received at least three doses of tetanus toxoid with the last dose < 5 years from the time of the injury.

17. Is the number of IPVs the crucial issue in determining if a child is up to date, or is it the spacing of these immunizations?

The spacing. The American Academy of Pediatrics recommends that a child receive three doses of IPV before the age of 18 months and a booster dose at the time of school entry. If a child does not keep up with this schedule and receives the third dose on or after the fourth birthday, a fourth IPV is not needed.

18. Is oral polio vaccine (OPV) given for routine immunization?

OPV no longer is recommended for routine immunization because of the risk of vaccine-associated paralytic polio from the excretion of the live virus in stool.

19. Should OPV ever be used?

Yes. There are a few instances when OPV may be needed:
- When mass vaccination is needed to control outbreaks of paralytic polio.
- When unimmunized children will be traveling to endemic areas before they are able to receive two doses of IPV spaced at least 6 weeks apart. Clinicians are encouraged to contact Traveler Clinics or the Centers for Disease Control to determine if polio is endemic to the family's travel destination.
- When parents refuse the appropriate number of injections to produce immunity. If OPV is used in this situation, it must be used only for the third and fourth dose.

20. Name important conditions that the pneumococcal vaccine (PCV-7) vaccine prevents.

If caused by *Streptococcus pneumoniae*, the following can be prevented:
Meningitis
Bacteremia
Pneumonia
Possibly otitis media

21. How many PCV-7 vaccinations are required?
The age at which vaccination is started determines the number of immunizations required.

AGE VACCINE STARTED	WHEN DOSES ARE GIVEN
2 mos	2, 4, 6, and 15 mos of age
4 mos	4, 6, 9, and 15 mos of age
6 mos	6, 9, 12, and 15 mos of age
9 mos	9, 12, and 15 mos of age
Between 12 and 24 mos	That visit and the next well-child visit
Between 2 and 5 years	One dose, depending on risk factors

22. What groups of children are at highest risk for pneumococcal disease?
Children with sickle cell disease, asplenia, dysfunctional spleen, and human immunodeficiency virus (HIV) infection.

23. Which children older than age 24 months are at high risk of contracting pneumococcal infection?
Children with chronic illnesses, such as congenital immune disorders, chronic cardiac conditions, chronic respiratory disease, chronic renal disease, and diabetes.

24. Which groups of children are at moderate risk of contracting pneumococcal disease?
• Children aged 2–3 years
• Children aged 3–5 years who are in out-of-home child care situations
• Children aged 3–5 years who are Native American, Alaskan, or African American

25. Which conditions put adolescents at high risk for pneumococcal disease?
Sickle cell disease, asplenia, nephrotic syndrome, cerebrospinal fluid leaks

26. For high-risk adolescents, is it better to use the 7-valent pneumococcal conjugate vaccine or the 23-valent polysaccharide vaccine?
The **23-valent vaccine** provides 80–90% of coverage in high-risk adolescents so it should not be replaced by the 7-valent vaccine, which provides only 50–60% of coverage against invasive disease in high-risk individuals. The 23-valent vaccine should be administered 5 years after the initial dose of the 23-valent vaccine.

27. What illnesses can infection with *H. influenzae* cause?
Common illnesses

Otitis media	Cellulitis
Sinusitis	Meningitis
Epiglottitis	Pneumonia
Septic arthritis	Empyema
Occult febrile bacteremia	

Less common illnesses

Purulent pericarditis	Osteomyelitis
Endocarditis	Peritonitis
Conjunctivitis	Glossitis

28. What change has brought about a decrease in the incidence of *H. influenzae* illnesses?
The introduction of the *H. influenzae* B (HIB) vaccine in the 1980s. Epiglottitis in particular has decreased in incidence.

29. Are there significant side effects from the HIB vaccine?

No. Adverse reactions are minimal and usually are localized to the site of the injection. The reactions may include pain, redness, and swelling at the site of the vaccination.

30. What side effects should the health care provider review with parents of a child receiving the 2-month group of DTaP, IPV, HIB, and PCV-7?

• Possibility of low-grade fever
• Irritability
• Soreness at the site of the DTaP and PCV-7 immunizations

31. What comfort measures can the nurse suggest to the caregivers of a child after the DTaP, IPV, HIB, and PVC-7 vaccines?

1. A dose of acetaminophen liquid, 15 mg/kg, given after these immunizations, then again in 4–6 hours helps to reduce pain at the site of the injection and to keep temperature within normal limits. This dose may be repeated five times in 24 hours if the infant is fussy and febrile.

2. A cold soak applied to the site of the DTaP and PCV-7 injections may help to reduce swelling in the first 24 hours after administration.

3. A warm soak at the site of these injections after the first 24 hours may help the vaccine to begin to be absorbed from the muscle.

32. Which immunizations should a 28-week preterm infant who is still in the newborn intensive care unit at 8 weeks of life receive?

The immunization schedule for preterm infants is the same as for full-term infants so the infant should receive DTaP, IPV, HIB, and PCV-7.

33. Should a preterm infant receive a hepatitis B vaccine?

Hepatitis B immunization should be started when the infant weighs at least 2 kg if the mother is not hepatitis B surface antigen positive at birth.

34. Which immunizations must be repeated if given even 1 day before the age of 12 months because of the potential decreased efficacy from circulating maternal antibodies?

MMR and Varivax.

35. Because the current MMR vaccine is derived from chick embryo tissue cultures, should egg-sensitive children be skin tested before the administration of the MMR?

Skin testing for these children is not recommended because the chick embryo cultures do not contain large amounts of egg cross-reacting proteins and because most reactions in egg-sensitive children after MMR are due to a reaction to other components of the vaccine, such as neomycin or gelatin, and not to the chick embryo tissue. However, children with anaphylactic response to eggs or questionable egg sensitivity are often referred to allergists for MMR administration.

36. Summarize the recommendations for the administration of the second MMR.

The second MMR must be given at least 1 month after the initial MMR. This brief interval between vaccines is needed in case of exposure to an active case of measles, mumps, or rubella. The second MMR typically is given between 4 and 6 years of age or in early adolescence.

37. Describe the possible adverse effects after immunization with varicella.

Side effects are generally mild and may include pain, redness, or swelling at the site of the injection. Some children may develop a generalized rash, whereas others develop a maculopapular or vesicular rash sometime within 1 month after vaccination.

38. What is the risk of transmission of varicella to contacts after immunization?

Transmission to contacts is rare and has occurred only when the vaccine recipient has developed a rash after immunization. Immunosuppressed contacts should be aware of this possibility and avoid contact with the rash.

39. How many doses of varicella vaccine are needed in a 15-year-old who has no documented varicella disease?

Two. The doses must be at least 1 month apart. If the interval between the first and second dose of Varivax is > 8 weeks, the recipient is susceptible to acquiring the natural disease.

40. Which groups of adolescents should not receive Varicella vaccine?

Immunocompromised adolescents, pregnant adolescents, and adolescents considering becoming pregnant in the following month.

41. What are the storage requirements for varicella vaccine?

1. The vaccine must be stored frozen at least − 15°C to maintain potency and efficacy.

2. A dose of reconstituted vaccine must be administered within 30 minutes of reconstitution with the diluent.

42. What are the most common routes of transmission of hepatitis B?
- Vertical transmission from an infected mother to her fetus
- Sexual contact with an infected individual
- Parenteral drug use
- Household contact with a carrier of hepatitis B
- Occupational exposure (e.g., needle stick, infected patients)

43. Discuss the current recommendation for immunization of infants born to hepatitis B–positive mothers?

Infants should receive hepatitis B virus **immunoglobulin** and the first dose of hepatitis B **vaccine** within 12 hours of birth. The second dose should be given 4 weeks later, and the final dose should be given at least by 6 months of age. The infant should be checked for immunity to hepatitis B after completing the series by having titers. If the infant is not yet immune, the series should be given again and immunity rechecked. If the infant still is not immune after completion of the second series of vaccines, no further effort is made.

44. Discuss the current recommendation for the spacing of hepatitis B vaccine.

The first dose of hepatitis B vaccine may be administered as soon after birth as possible in infants weighing > 2 kg or anytime thereafter. The second dose must be administered at least 4 weeks from the first dose, and the third dose must be administered at least 2 months from dose 2 and at least 4 months from dose 1. If the series is started in early infancy, the infant must be at least 6 months old before the third dose is administered.

45. What is Recombivax HB?

This hepatitis vaccine provides protection for adolescents with only two doses instead of the usual three doses given to infants. This recombinant vaccine was developed in an effort to promote complete protection because many adolescents do not return for the series of three immunizations. The concentration of Recombivax is 10 µg/1.0 mL instead of 5 µg/0.5 mL that is used in the three-dose series. The second dose of Recombivax is administered 4 months from the first. Immunity is found to be the same as the three-dose regimen.

46. Summarize the current recommendations for administration of hepatitis A vaccine.

It is recommended for children and adolescents in some states that have a high prevalence rate of hepatitis A, and it is recommended for high-risk individuals.

47. Identify individuals at high risk for hepatitis A.
- Individuals traveling to countries where the disease is endemic
- Intravenous drug users
- Individuals with clotting factor disorders
- Individuals with chronic liver disease
- Individuals working with primates

48. What are the current recommendations for the use of palivizumab (Synagis) or respiratory syncytial virus (RSV) prophylaxis?

Palivizumab generally is recommended for the prevention of RSV infection in susceptible infants < 24 months old (infants born at < 35 weeks' gestation and infants with chronic lung disease. The vaccine is administered monthly at 15 mg/kg throughout the RSV season (usually November to April) depending on the local epidemiology of the virus. Some children with significant lung disease may benefit from RSV prophylaxis for two seasons.

Because of the expense of the product, use of this vaccine should be limited to infants born between 32 and 35 weeks' gestation with the following additional risk factors:
- Several younger siblings
- Attendance at day care
- Exposure to tobacco smoke in the home
- Anticipated cardiac surgery
- Distance to and availability of hospital care for severe respiratory illness

49. Which groups of children and adolescents should receive influenza vaccine?

Patients with chronic respiratory or cardiac disease, diabetes mellitus, renal dysfunction, hemoglobinopathies, immunosuppressive disorders, or long-term aspirin therapies. Declining immunity a year after vaccination and different viral strains each year make it necessary to be immunized yearly with the current vaccine.

50. Is it ever necessary to give two doses of influenza vaccine?

Yes. In children younger than 9 years old who are receiving the vaccine for the first time, two doses must be administered 1 month apart.

51. Is the concurrent use of steroids a problem when thinking about giving a child the influenza vaccine?

Probably not. Low-dose steroids or brief periods of steroid use do not interfere with a child's ability to mount an immune response to influenza vaccine. Extended use of high-dose steroids may weaken the antibody response so that influenza immunization should be deferred during the time of steroid administration if it does not interfere with the start of the influenza season.

52. Is it safe to administer influenza vaccine to children who are egg sensitive?

No. The influenza vaccine is derived from egg protein, and children who have anaphylactoid reactions to eggs should not receive influenza immunization because the risk of anaphylaxis is too great and because the influenza vaccine is needed yearly, putting the child at risk too often.

53. What about children who have local allergic reactions to eggs?

Local allergic reactions to eggs or feathers are not contraindications to influenza vaccine.

54. Which vaccine has recently has been recommended for all college freshmen living in dormitories to consider?

Meningococcal vaccine because it has been noted that college freshmen living in dormitories have a higher than expected prevalence rate of meningococcal disease.

55. What is the biggest drawback to the use of the meningococcal vaccine?

It may provide a false sense of security because it does not provide protection against serogroup B, which causes one third of meningococcal disease. Recipients should be informed of this fact when getting the vaccine.

56. When is a rabies vaccine indicated?

Rabies vaccination is recommended after a bite by any animal that has a high likelihood of being rabid or after contamination of mucous membranes or exposed tissue by a possibly rabid animal. **High-risk animals** include raccoons, skunks, bats, and foxes. Coyotes, cattle, dogs, cats, and ferrets are less likely to be rabid. Management of possible rabies exposure is done best with the collaboration of local epidemiologists and infectious disease specialists who are aware of local risks. At-risk patients receive initial treatment with rabies immunoglobulin based on body weight, then a series of rabies vaccines (1 mL/dose) given on the first day of exposure prophylaxis, then on days 3, 7, 14, and 28.

57. What is BCG vaccine?

Bacille Calmette-Guérin (BCG) is a live vaccine that is used in 100 countries worldwide to try to prevent serious manifestations of *Mycobacterium tuberculosis*. It does not prevent infection with this bacillus, however.

58. Discuss the implications of use of BCG vaccine.

BCG currently is not recommended for general use in the United States, but many immigrant children may have received this vaccination in infancy in their country of origin. Careful and individualized interpretation of subsequent **tuberculin skin tests** must be done in a child who received BCG. Interpretation is based on age at receiving BCG, the possibility of multiple injections with BCG, risk factors, and underlying health.

59. What are the current recommendations for immunizing children adopted from overseas?

Children adopted from overseas by families in the United States should be immunized according to the currently recommended schedule used in the United States. If there is any doubt about the written records received from overseas, such as age at which vaccines were administered, interval between doses, number of doses, or immunogenicity of the vaccine, titers should be obtained or the immunizations should be readministered. Children adopted from orphanages in some countries in Eastern Europe and some countries in Asia may come to the United States with inaccurate records or having received less potent vaccines than recommended here. It is up to the caregiver to decide, but it is better to overimmunize a child than to underimmunize.

60. Discuss specific recommendations for the immunization of immunosuppressed children.

Recommendations are based on the degree and nature of each child's immunosuppression and his or her susceptibility to infection. **Primary immunodeficiencies** often are inherited or congenital, whereas **secondary immunodeficiencies** develop as the result of other illnesses, such as malignancy, HIV, or organ transplantation. Because there is such heterogeneity within these groups of children and because immune status may change with disease treatment, vaccine administration must be individualized.

BIBLIOGRAPHY

1. American Academy of Pediatrics. Available at www.aap.org.
2. Centers for Disease Control and Prevention: Recommendation of the Advisory Committee on Immunization Practices (ACIP). MMWR Morb Mortal Wkly Rep. Available at www.cdc. gov/nip/publications/ACIP-list.htm.
3. Centers for Disease Control and Prevention: Immunization of adolescents: Recommendations of the Advisory Committee on Immunization Practices, the American Academy of Pediatrics, the American Academy of Family Physicians, and the American Medical Association. MMWR Morb Mortal Wkly Rep 45:1–16, 1996.
4. Centers for Disease Control and Prevention: Recommended childhood immunization schedule: United States 2001. MMWR Morb Mortal Wkly Rep 50:7–10, 19, 2001.
5. Dias M, Marcuse E: When parents resist immunizations. Contemp Pediatr 17:75–86, 2000.
6. Edwards K, Thombs D: The new pneumococcal vaccine: What practitioners need to know. Contemp Pediatr (suppl) 17:3–15, 2000.
7. Humiston S, Strikas R: Routine childhood vaccination update: Educating the office staff. Pediatr Ann 30:329–341, 2001.
8. Pickering L (ed): Red Book 2000: Report of the Committee on Infectious Diseases, 25th ed. Elk Grove Village, IL, American Academy of Pediatrics, 2000.
9. Santole J, Szilagyi P, Rodewald L: Barriers to immunization and missed opportunities. Pediatr Ann 27:366–374, 1998.
10. Snyder R: Recommendations for storing and handling vaccines. Pediatr Ann 30:346–348, 2001.

17. ADOLESCENCE AND REPRODUCTIVE HEALTH

Linda J. Allan Pasto, MS, RN

1. Define adolescence.

To grow into maturity. Adolescence encompasses the second largest period of growth during a life span.

2. What period of time encompasses adolescence?

Adolescence generally is considered to cover the period beginning with the development of secondary sex characteristics at ages 11–13 and ending with full physical growth at ages 18–20.

Another view of adolescence includes the period of secondary education through the completion of college—ages 13–21.

3. How is the adolescent period characterized?

1. Early adolescence   Ages 11–14
2. Middle adolescence   Ages 15–17
3. Late adolescence   Ages 18–21

4. Do boys and girls mature at the same rate?

Generally, girls start maturing faster than boys, although boys catch up before the end of high school.

5. What are the physical changes that occur in girls?

Hormone levels increase until about 3 years after menstruation begins, when they peak and remain at that level throughout the reproductive years. The first indication of the onset of puberty is the appearance of breast buds. The initial menstruation usually occurs about 2 years after these first physical changes.

6. What is the usual sequence of maturational changes in girls?

1. Breast changes
2. Rapid increase in height and weight
3. Growth of pubic hair
4. Appearance of axillary hair
5. Menstruation (first time referred to as menarche)
6. Abrupt deceleration of growth

7. What are the physical changes that occur in boys?

Similar to in girls, the changes are initiated by an increase in hormone levels. The first change is testicular enlargement.

8. List the usual sequence of maturational changes in boys.

1. Testicular enlargement
2. Growth of pubic hair, axillary hair, hair on upper lip, hair on face, and hair elsewhere on the body
3. Penile enlargement
4. Rapid height increase
5. Changes in the larynx and deepening of the voice
6. Nocturnal emissions
7. Abrupt deceleration of growth

9. Describe the expected growth and development during the early adolescent period.

This is a period of rapid growth and many body changes. Girls are generally taller and slightly heavier than boys. They appear awkward and gangly as growth occurs. Secondary sex characteristics appear, which are a cause for comparison and concern. Self-consciousness and low self-esteem are common. There is conformity to group norms. Individuals seek peer group affiliations to deal with the instability generated by the rapid changes occurring to each individual.

Wide mood swings, daydreaming, angry outbursts, limited abstract thinking, and frequent self-comparisons with peers are common. Rebellious behavior begins, because of the struggle over independence and dependence issues.

10. What are the physical characteristics of the middle adolescent period?
- Physical growth rapidly decreases for girls, while it continues to accelerate in boys.
- Acne peaks and sweat gland functions increase.
- Dental problems (malocclusions) occur in 50% of teens by this time.
- Movement becomes more coordinated, and physical endurance increases.

11. Discuss the emotional and psychological characteristics of the middle adolescent period.

Adolescents tend to be self-centered, moody, narcissistic, and intensely private. Idealism characterizes their thinking. This is a difficult period for parents because there are major conflicts over independence and control. There is a great push for emancipation. Peers take on a central role with acceptance by peers being of paramount importance. Pairing off into couples is experimented with during this time. There is a strong need to establish identity and affirm self-image. Communication is difficult because there is a tendency to withdraw when upset and to have difficulty asking for help.

12. Describe the characteristics of the late adolescent period.

Physical growth is almost complete by this time. Body image and gender role are established. There is a comfort with physical growth and body changes and stable self-esteem. Adolescents are less emotionally labile. Abstract thinking is well ensconced. Future plans are often a topic of discussion and include educational and vocational goals. The social group is less dominant because pairing off is common. Separation from parents on a physical and emotional plane is mostly complete. This period represents an easing of conflicts between parent and child, evolving into an adult relationship. Family ties are maintained, although there is independence.

13. What other physical changes occur in adolescence?
- Heart and lungs continue to increase in size and capacity.
- Blood volume and systolic blood pressure increase; pulse rate, respiratory rate, and basal metabolic rate decrease.
- Senses continue to develop, especially smell.
- Hearing peaks at age 13, whereas touch and sight are fully mature at this point.

14. What does Erikson identify as the developmental stage of adolescence?

Development of a **sense of identity versus role diffusion**. This is initiated first through a group identity in which teenagers can explore differences between themselves and their parents. They seek to be different from their parents through dress, fads, language, and interests. Individual identity is difficult and needs to include the incorporation of the body changes that are occurring into the adolescent's self-concept.

15. Describe the changes in cognitive development that Piaget identifies.

Piaget's final stage of formal operations produces **abstract thinking**. Adolescents are able to think in a future orientation. They use logic in their thought processes and can manipulate more than two types of variables at one time. They are able to look at and explore their own thinking and that of others. It is a time of exploration of personal philosophies, future planning, and goal setting.

16. What changes occur in adolescent social development?

Peers become an increasingly significant influence in adolescent lives. The peer group provides support, a sense of belonging, and a feeling of strength and collective power.

Although **parents** remain a primary influence in teenaged lives, relationships change as the individual seeks more independence. Behavior exhibited by the adolescent toward the parent is triggered by the struggle for independence and external boundaries and restrictions placed by the parents.

17. What are the most common areas for struggle between adolescents and parents?

Dress	Friendships	Telephone use
Language	Dating	Time commitments
Curfews	Homework	Cars
Money	Chores	Drinking and drugs

18. What forms of sexual expression are expected during adolescence?

Individual masturbation	Oral and anal sex
Petting	Sexual intercourse
Mutual masturbation	

19. What role do peers play in adolescent sexual expression?

Peers provide pressure to each other to conform to group behavior, which may include sexual activity.

20. Is homosexuality expressed in adolescence?

Yes. The adolescent period is when gay, lesbian, and bisexual individuals become aware of same-sex attractions.

21. What are the risks of homosexuality for the adolescent?

Homosexual adolescents are at increased risk for risk-taking behaviors because of society's reaction to their sexual expression. They are more at risk for:

Suicidal ideation	Running away from home
Suicide attempts	Drug and alcohol use

22. Name the major causes of morbidity in adolescence.

Acquired immunodeficiency syndrome (AIDS)
Sexually transmitted diseases (STDs), especially *Chlamydia*
Pregnancy
Depression
Violence
Injury

23. How can risk-taking behaviors be reduced?

Listen, listen, listen, and respect! Reduction of risk-taking behaviors can be accomplished by empowering adolescents to take charge of their health through education and skill building and working on improving self-esteem. Adolescents need information and caring and respectful professionals who listen and allow adolescents to make decisions for themselves.

24. What should health care providers know regarding confidentiality?

In many states, minors can receive education and treatment without parental consent. Many states mandate confidentiality for substance abuse and sex-related issues. The exceptions to this mandate are if the minor is suicidal, has experienced child abuse, or is threatening homicide. The adolescent needs to know these parameters before confidentiality is assured.

25. How can a trusting relationship be established with an adolescent?

When ground rules have been established, including confidentiality and honesty, getting teens to talk is the next challenge. The least personal questions should be presented first. Asking questions that can be answered easily allows the teen to feel important and not "stupid." These questions could be about school, normal activities, and previous health care. Then, questions on topics such as smoking, substance and alcohol use, and sexuality can follow. With sensitive issues, questions should be approached in a nonthreatening manner. For example, a question can be prefaced by stating that many adolescents worry about the particular issue or that it is common for an adolescent to experience this; the ask: "Have you ever worried about this issue?" Teens needs to be praised for any healthy behavior they currently are following.

26. Discuss the nutritional needs of adolescents.

Adolescents need to have an understanding of the **Food Guide Pyramid** and the relationship between food intake, activity, health status, and weight. Food sources to increase intake of calcium, iron, and other important minerals and vitamins are vital topics of discussion. Guidance in choosing low-fat, high-fiber options should be included in information given. Adolescents who choose a vegetarian lifestyle need careful assistance to ensure their diets contain all essential components.

27. Why do adolescents have problems meeting their nutritional needs?
- Adolescents are influenced by **peers** in their eating habits.
- Meals often are eaten away from home, so family influence is diminished.
- Time is a factor, and meals are eaten quickly or skipped.
- Meals often are lacking in fresh fruits and vegetables, especially those that are high in ascorbic acid.
- **Milk** consumption drops in favor of soft or sport drinks. Regular intake of calcium-rich foods is critical for future health for males and females.
- **Snacks** are chosen more for convenience than nutritional value.

28. List three health problems associated with nutrition.
1. Obesity
2. Anorexia nervosa
3. Bulimia

29. What are the causes of obesity?

Poor dietary habits and sedentary lifestyle.

30. How can nutrition issues be addressed to adolescents?
- Adolescents need to be encouraged to eat snacks that are nutritious. Nutritious snacks should be made readily available.
- Review of nutritional information and balanced diets should be included in health classes and provided by school dietitians.
- Obese teens need to have an integrated approach to their treatment that includes regular exercise, behavioral therapy, support group involvement with peers, and education.

31. What is anorexia nervosa?

This eating disorder is characterized by:
- Refusal to maintain adequate body weight
- Preoccupation with and fear of obesity
- Amenorrhea
- Feelings of inadequacy
- Physical symptoms, such as lanugo, fatigue, dull hair, dry skin, and muscle wasting

32. How is bulimia characterized?

Bulimia presents as recurrent episodes of binge eating that may be followed by episodes of purging either through forced vomiting or laxative use. Other methods to avoid weight gain include excessive exercising, use of diuretics, and fasting. Bulimia also includes an excessive and persistent overconcern with body image.

33. How are anorexia nervosa and bulimia treated?

A thorough **medical examination** determines any serious effects of improper nutritional intake. Many individuals also suffer from depression or other psychiatric disorders. Resistance to treatment is common so that many disciplines must be involved in the treatment. **Hospitalization** may be required to achieve physiologic stability. Monitoring of intake and output, vital signs, electrolytes, and cardiac status is crucial. A dietitian's involvement is helpful in planning gradual weight gain. Risk for suicide must be evaluated and observed for and any evidence of denial, trickery, or resistance to weight gain. **Contracts** for behavior are implemented as the teen is involved in a day treatment program. The family must be involved in the treatment plan to ensure the highest level of success.

34. Why do adolescents need to be counseled about osteoporosis?

Adequate calcium intake is important because calcium stores established during adolescence can help prevent osteoporosis in later life for males and females. Teen girls should be counseled to avoid excessive cola intake because cola contains phosphorus, which interferes with calcium intake.

35. What general health care concerns should the nurse have for adolescents?

Adolescents need to have health promotion and disease prevention provided for them even if they seem to resist or refuse. They need to be encouraged to take more responsibility for their health as they increase their independence from their parents.

36. What are the major health care concerns in adolescents?

Sleep and rest	Immunizations
Exercise and activity	Sexuality
Safety	Skin care
Dental care	Reduction of risk-taking behaviors

37. How much sleep do adolescents need?

Adolescents need to be encouraged to get adequate sleep and rest to promote proper growth and development. Teenagers require at least **8 hours of sleep**. They may experience more difficulty waking in the morning. They are apt to stay up later as hormones change their daily sleep-wake clock. School studies may force later bedtimes because activities crowd available time.

38. What can schools do to accommodate adolescents' changing sleep and rest needs?

Some schools across the United States are changing their start times to reflect the adolescent's shifting sleep-wake cycles, which have an impact on learning, especially early in the day.

39. List immunization needs for adolescents.

- A second measles, mumps, and rubella (MMR) vaccine may be needed if not already administered.
- Tetanus booster is required every 10 years.
- Hepatitis B vaccine is suggested for adolescents before they become sexually active.
* Varicella vaccine is needed if there is no history of chickenpox.

40. Summarize health screening recommendations.

- Vision screening should be done annually because refractive problems surface during adolescence, and glasses or contact lenses may be required.
- Blood pressure should be monitored as a screen for hypertension.

- Height, weight, and body mass index tracking could highlight growth problems and eating disorders.
- Laboratory values, including hemoglobin, hematocrit, and urinalysis, should be obtained to rule out various diseases, such as anemia.

41. What should teens know about illness prevention?
Teens should be taught the importance of:
Testicular and breast self-examination
Routine physical examinations
Routine dental checkups
Regular vision screening
Regular gynecologic examinations for sexually active females

42. Are there specific concerns for teens and physical activity?
Yes. As the cardiovascular system continues to grow and mature, physical activities must be matched to the adolescent's endurance. Adolescents may fatigue easily with activity and must be accorded periods of rest.

Because regular exercise is an important part of a person's overall health, teens should be encouraged to try different forms of activities and plan daily exercise. Parents need to evaluate an exercise program for safety, rest, fluid intake, cardiovascular fitness, and psychological well-being. During the period of growth spurt, extra care needs to be taken to ensure maximal health.

Self-esteem can be improved through participation in physical exercise and activities. Guidance should be provided regarding prevention of sports injuries and common problems to watch for. Proper use of protective devices, such as eye wear and shin guards, can prevent injuries from occurring.

43. What is overuse syndrome?
A syndrome caused by repetitive trauma to a particular structure when the same movements are performed over and over. It results in inflammation of involved structures, pain, swelling, tenderness, and possible disability.

44. Give examples of overuse syndrome.
Stress fractures
Tennis elbow
Osgood-Schlatter disease

45. How is overuse syndrome treated?
Rest of the affected structure, which means decreased activity and alternative exercise
Cold therapy
Taping
Bracing
Splinting
Nonsteroidal anti-inflammatory drugs to treat inflammation

46. What dental needs are specific to adolescents?
- Regular checkups should be obtained every 6 months.
- Adolescents need to be reminded to brush and floss twice daily to prevent caries.
- Nutritional guidance to avoid diets high in sweets and alternative snacks should be included in yearly care.
- Adolescence is often the time when braces are applied, which has implications for body image and oral hygiene.

47. Should adolescents receive fluoride supplements?
Fluoride supplements should be provided in areas of nonfluoridated water.

48. Define acne.

An inflammatory disease of the skin involving sebaceous glands and hair follicles. It can lead to physical and emotional scarring.

49. How many teens actually experience acne?

85%.

50. What causes acne?

The cause is unknown, but it is triggered by **hormonal influences** and **stress**. Foods traditionally were thought to play a role in outbreaks, but they no longer are considered culprits.

51. How is acne treated?

Treatment is geared toward prevention of scarring and promotion of a positive body image. **Topical medications**, adequate rest, adequate fluid intake, and use of sunscreen are part of the usual treatment plan. Oral antibiotics such as **tetracycline** may be used in cases of severe inflammation. Hygiene measures, such as regular hair and skin washing and avoidance of placing hands on the face, need to be taught. Because it takes weeks before medications are effective, adolescents need encouragement to continue treatment.

52. What are the health implications of body piercing and tattooing?

Adolescents need to be careful to have procedures performed under sterile conditions. They need to understand signs of infection, bleeding complications, allergies to products used, and scarring. Tattoos should be considered a permanent process. Although removal is possible, it is difficult and expensive. Impulse decisions to obtain a tattoo may be made under the influence of peer pressure, alcohol, or drugs. Blood-borne infections are a risk anytime the skin is penetrated

53. Is sun tanning a concern for teens?

Yes. Sun tanning is a health risk, which may result in skin cancer later in life. Teens need to understand the cumulative effect of sun exposure and how to minimize their risks. Use of tanning beds for year-round tans increases the cumulative effect of UV rays. The use of sunscreens, hats, and protective clothing is helpful. Teens should be cautioned about sun exposure if they are taking any medication, such as some acne treatments, that may be potentiated by UV light.

54. Why is sexuality an area of concern?

Adolescents are bombarded by sexual messages from the media beginning at an early age. They are pressured by society to date, and hormonal influences urge them toward experimentation. Misinformation is common because teens often get their sex education from peers, media, movies, television, and magazines.

55. What topics should be covered when educating teens about sexuality?
  • Normal body changes and emotional responses
  • STDs
  • Birth control
  • Pregnancy and childbirth
  • Typical health problems, such as amenorrhea, dysmenorrhea, vaginitis, endometriosis, gynecomastia, and varicoceles
  • Alternative sexual expressions
  • Safe sex
  • Dealing with peer pressure

56. How effective is abstinence-based education?

Abstinence-only programs have not been found to be effective. Teens need more comprehensive information to make informed decisions.

57. When should birth control information be given to teens?

Girls are likely to be sexually active 6–12 months before seeking birth control measures, so proactive education is crucial. Thus, girls and boys should be given information when they are preteens so that later they can make informed decisions.

58. What risk factors contribute to adolescent pregnancy?

Low self-esteem	Lack of parental support
Academic failure	Family history of early pregnancy
Low socioeconomic status, especially poverty	Peer pressure
	A hopeless outlook on the future
History of sexual abuse	

59. What factors should be considered in selecting a contraception method?
- The individual's cognitive level
- The individual's physical and mental health
- The individual's ability to understand directions
- Communication with partner
- Frequency of intercourse
- Motivation of both partners
- Access to health care and insurance
- Finances
- Commitment to use of birth control
- Comfort with body
- Number and gender of partners

60. Which three types of birth control are teens most likely to choose?

(1) Withdrawal, (2) condoms, and (3) oral contraceptive pills.

61. Which other type of birth control is increasing in use among adolescents?

Injectable contraceptives, such as medroxyprogesterone acetate (Depo-Provera).

62. What is risk taking?

Risk taking is considered to be part of normal growth and development for the adolescent. The resultant behavior may increase self-confidence and enable self-exploration, such as learning to snowboard. Alternatively, it may put the adolescent's health and life at risk, as in the use of firearms or performance-enhancing drugs.

63. What are some common risk-taking behaviors?

Having sex without using birth control
Driving under the influence of drugs or alcohol
Experimenting with firearms
Skate boarding or inline skating (Rollerblades)

64. How should risk-taking behaviors and injury prevention addressed?

Discussion and assessment of risk-taking behaviors and injury prevention should occur at every encounter with the adolescent, whether it is during a sports or well-child visit or during an acute care visit if it is applicable. Health promotion activities also can be part of school or sports programs.

65. How many adolescents are affected by depression?

59% (depending on the type of population).

66. What signs are indicative of adolescent depression?

Fatigue	Suicidal ideation or attempts
Difficulty sleeping	Physical complaints with no physical cause

Significant weight loss or gain
Loss of energy
Feelings of worthlessness or helplessness

Decreased ability to concentrate or think
Irritability or agitation

67. What information should the nurse include in the initial assessment of a depressed teen?
The nurse should record the teen's history in the following areas:

Mood
Suicidal ideation or plan
Triggers to depressive periods
Recent stressors

Family structure and environment
Physiologic symptoms
Daily activities

68. What specific questions should the nurse ask during assessment for depression?
1. Do you feel sad often?
2. Do you ever feel life is not worth living?
3. Have you ever thought about hurting or killing yourself?

69. What is the usual treatment for depression?
Based on the information gathered in the assessment, treatment may include **antidepressant** or related drugs and counseling for the individual and family. **Hospitalization** may be required initially so that specialized care can be provided. Specific changes in the environment often need to be implemented to allow a teen to have a sense of control. Teachers and parents should be educated about depression because they are likely to be the first to notice symptoms.

70. What clues may indicate that an adolescent is considering suicide?
1. Notes that are vague but include a goodbye or leaving theme and giving away possessions.
2. Sudden changes in behavior, especially calmness, after a history of anxiety or agitation
3. Statements made about suicide or self-harm
4. Preoccupation with death
5. History of sexual or physical abuse
6. Frequent risk-taking or abusive behavior (e.g., excessive use of drugs or alcohol, sexually promiscuous, running away from home, stealing, vandalism)
7. Overwhelming sense of shame, guilt, or self-doubt
8. Signs of mental illness, such as severe depression, hallucinations, or delusions
9. Significant life event, such as breakup of a relationship or death of family member
10. Loss of energy and loss of interest in daily activities
11. Changes in sleeping pattern or appetite
12. Physical complaints, such as stomachaches and headaches
13. Sudden change in school performance
14. Flat or dull affect, remaining distant from others, and social withdrawal
15. Family history of suicide or previous history of attempt

71. How can suicide be prevented?
• Identifying individuals at risk can allow for intervention before an attempt is successful.
• Screening for depression helps get support to teens who need it. Teens should be asked if they have suicidal thoughts if signs of depression are present.
• Peers should be encouraged to report or ask for help when friends even mention the thought of suicide.
• Providing education at the middle school and high school level gives information about signs and services and reduces the social stigma.
• Providing support after a suicide can help prevent more incidents because it is common for suicides to cluster in a community.
• No threats or gestures should ever be ignored because that individual usually is asking for help.

• The lethality and potentiality of the threat or plan need to be assessed to determine how well developed the suicide plan is.

72. What should be done for a teen who threatens suicide?

If the adolescent has a specific plan, he or she must be monitored carefully at all times. The adolescent must not have access to firearms, belts, drugs (over-the-counter and prescription), scarves, shoestrings, sharp objects, matches, or lighters. A threat should be taken seriously, and measures should be implemented to ensure the adolescent's safety.

73. List the signs and symptoms of mononucleosis.

Early signs	Later signs
Headache	Fever
Chills	Sore throat
Malaise	Pharyngitis
Fatigue	Splenomegaly
Low-grade fever	Cervical adenopathy
Loss of appetite	

74. How is mononucleosis diagnosed?

The Monospot test is used most commonly.

75. Is mononucleosis really spread by kissing?

It can be. Mononucleosis, which is caused by the Epstein-Barr virus, is transmitted through saliva, close intimate contact, and blood. Although it can be spread by kissing, there are many other ways to contract the virus.

76. Can an adolescent with mononucleosis still participate in sports?

Some sports. Care must be taken during the recovery period to avoid trauma to the spleen because it may be enlarged and at risk for rupture. Contact sports, such as football and soccer, are not recommended. Noncontact sports, such as swimming, can be continued if energy levels are sufficient.

77. Describe the treatment for mononucleosis.

When the diagnosis is confirmed, rest and treatment of symptoms by simple remedies are implemented. Normal routines can resume when tolerance of activity is achieved. Acute symptoms usually disappear in 7–10 days; fatigue may linger for 2–4 weeks.

78. Is asthma a health care problem for teens?

Yes. Asthma is a major chronic health problem of adolescence. Adolescents who have been diagnosed with asthma in childhood are at risk for **noncompliance**. They may be reluctant to admit they have a health problem or choose to ignore warning signs of an approaching attack. **Sports involvement** may exacerbate the problem unless coaches are supportive of the athlete's needs. Risk-taking behaviors can compound the problem if asthmatic adolescents start **cigarette smoking**.

79. Asthma is a leading cause of school absences. What can be done to avoid unnecessary missed days and prevent attacks?

• Teens need to have access to health care and medications.
• Teens should have knowledge of warning signs. Early recognition helps prevent unnecessary hospitalizations.
• Teens should be aware of environmental triggers that initiate their attacks.
• If asthma is induced by **exercise**, preventive measures need to be instituted before exercise is begun.
• **Viruses** are the most common trigger of asthma, so exposure to individuals who are ill should be avoided.

• Teens should monitor their air exchange using a peak flowmeter, which empowers teens with some control over their asthma.

80. Is teen pregnancy still a problem?

Yes. Although pregnancy rates have dropped during the last decade, many teens still become pregnant each year. Although the mortality rate for teens has decreased, the morbidity rate remains high.

81. If a teen is not using birth control, how long will it take before she becomes pregnant?

Approximately 80% of teen pregnancies occur within **1 year of initiating intercourse**; approximately 20% of pregnancies occur in the first month.

82. What are the health risks of adolescent pregnancy?

Pregnant teens are at increased for:

Pregnancy-induced hypertension	Low–birth-weight infants
Cephalopelvic disproportion	Premature infants
Preterm labor	Intrauterine growth retardation
Prolonged labor	Neonatal mortality
Iron-deficiency anemia	

83. What are the major social consequences of adolescent pregnancy?

Failure to complete schooling
Social isolation

84. When should an adolescent girl have her first pelvic examination?

The first examination should occur by age 18 or when the teen has become sexually active. Examinations should be done annually and may need to be more frequent depending on risk factors.

85. Which risk factors should warrant more frequent pelvic examinations?

Presence of an STD	History of sexual health problems
A partner who has an STD	Unusual vaginal or pelvic pain
A new sex partner or multiple partners	Abnormal vaginal discharge or bleeding
Plans to become pregnant	Painful intercourse

86. What should the gynecologic examination include?

1. Medical and reproductive history
2. Blood pressure, weight, and urine sample
3. A short physical examination, assessing the heart, lungs, skin, throat, and breasts
4. A vaginal examination to examine reproductive structures and the vaginal areas for signs of infection
5. A Papanicolaou (Pap) smear while examining the cervix
6. STD testing if a teen is sexually active

87. Why are STDs such a health risk for teens?

The type of cells that make up an adolescent's cervix are more susceptible to STDs, especially **human papillomavirus** and *Chlamydia*. The adolescent's immune system has not been exposed to these organisms, so resistance has not developed yet. Teens also are less likely to seek medical treatment if they are concerned about parental knowledge or involvement.

88. Name the most common STD that affects teens.

Chlamydia.

89. What is pelvic inflammatory disease?

Pelvic inflammatory disease (PID) is an infection of the upper genital tract, often caused by untreated STDs, especially gonorrhea and *Chlamydia*. It may lead to life-threatening infection or future infertility.

90. Why is pelvic inflammatory disease a concern for adolescents?

Teens account for 20% of all PID cases. Teens may not be aware of signs and symptoms of STDs and may not have access to health care services for treatment.

91. How does sexual assault affect the adolescent population?

- The incidence of sexual assault (rape) is significantly higher for teens and young adults than any other population.
- Date or acquaintance rape is a growing problem.
- Use of alcohol or recreational drugs increases the risk for rape to happen.
- Other risk factors include young age at first sexual activity, early age of first menarche, history of sexual abuse, developmental disability, and homosexual identification.

92. Summarize the treatment for a rape victim.

1. **Information** needs to be obtained regarding details of the rape, including time, location, date, and other related factors.

2. A **vaginal examination** is performed to gather forensic evidence, such as semen, blood, pubic hairs, evidence of trauma, and blood to test for STDs, especially gonorrhea and human immunodeficiency virus (HIV). Victims should be told not to bathe or shower before the examination is completed. The examination should be done with a woman present for support.

3. **Prophylactic penicillin** may be prescribed.

4. **Pregnancy prevention** with high-dose estrogen is offered if the teen is not pregnant or using hormone-based contraceptives.

5. **Follow-up care** is needed to observe for possible STDs and to provide referrals for emotional support through victims' advocate programs, crisis intervention, and counseling.

93. Is smoking an issue for teens?

Yes. Adolescent smoking is a major health issue with approximately 3000 teens taking up smoking every day. Although 75% of teens desire to quit, most health education programs are aimed at prevention rather than treatment.

94. What are effective approaches to helping teens stop smoking?

Because teens are image focused, strategies that address immediate **effects on appearance** are considered to be the most effective. The tobacco smell on the breath and nicotine stains on teeth and fingers should be pointed out. The physiologic vasoconstrictive effect of nicotine on **athletic performance** should be presented.

BIBLIOGRAPHY

1. Allard-Hendren R: Alcohol use and adolescent pregnancy. J Matern Child Nurs 25:159–162, 2000.
2. Ashwill JW, Droske SC: Nursing Care of Children: Principles and Practice. Philadelphia, W.B. Saunders, 1997.
3. Fritz DJ: Adolescent smoking cessation: How effective have we been? J Pediatr Nurs 15:299–306, 2000.
4. Lesser J: Health-related problems in a vulnerable population: Pregnant teens and adolescent mothers. Nurs Clin North Am 34:289–299, 2000.
5. Muscari ME: Adolescent health: The first gynecologic exam. Am J Nurs 99:66–68, 1999.
6. Muscari ME: Prevention: Are we really reaching today's teens? J Matern Child Nurs 24:87–91, 1999.

18. THE CHILD IN THE CRITICAL CARE UNIT

Lauren R. Sorce, RN, MSN, CCRN, CPNP,
Andrea Kline, RN, MS, CCRN, PCCNP, *and Joyce Weishaar*, RN, MSN, CCNS

SEDATION AND PAIN MANAGEMENT

1. What is conscious sedation?

A minimally depressed level of consciousness in which the child is able to maintain the airway independently and respond to physical stimulation and verbal commands. This type of sedation generally is used for procedures that produce anxiety, discomfort, or pain or that are lengthy and require a child to remain still.

2. List examples of procedures for which conscious sedation could be used.

Placement of a peripherally inserted central line   Laceration repair
Lumbar puncture   Magnetic resonance imaging
Fracture reduction   Computed tomography

3. What is deep sedation?

A controlled state of depressed consciousness or unconsciousness from which the child is not easily aroused. The child may lose protective reflexes and be unable to protect the airway independently.

4. List examples of procedures for which deep sedation could be used.

Cardiac catheterization
Endoscopy with biopsy
Polyp removal

5. How is the agent for sedation and analgesia selected?

The selection of an agent depends on the child's condition, current medical problems, current medications, drug allergies, and medical history. Generally, if the child is experiencing **anxiety**, a **sedative** may be used. The best drug for the child is that which is available, easy to administer, acts rapidly, lasts for the period of time during which the child will be anxious (during the procedure), and has a rapid recovery. If the child is experiencing **pain**, an **analgesic agent** may be used. Sedative agents usually lack analgesic properties, and analgesic agents may lack sedative properties. The selection of the appropriate medication should be determined on an individual basis.

6. What scales are available to assess pain in a critically ill child?

Self-reporting scales and observational scales. **Self-reporting scales** rely on the child to report his or her pain. Examples are rank order of pain on a scale of 1 to 10 and pointing to the painful area on a doll. **Observational scales** rely on the assessor to determine the level of pain depending on the scale used. Examples are the FACES scale, the Oucher scale, and the FLACC scale. Each element of the scale is scored and pain level is determined.

7. When are neuromuscular blocking agents used?

- During procedures (intubation and surgery)
- To facilitate mechanical ventilation and oxygenation
- To reduce oxygen consumption

- To stabilize cardiovascular status
- To reduce increased intracranial pressure (ICP)
- To maintain metabolic balance
- To eliminate shivering and striated muscle hyperactivity
- To immobilize extremities for patient safety

8. Discuss key issues in caring for the child receiving neuromuscular blocking agents.

Neuromuscular blocking agents *do not* provide sedation or analgesia. Sedation or analgesia *must* be administered concurrently when using neuromuscular blocking agents; otherwise the child experiences complete awareness of his or her surroundings but is unable to move, speak, or respond. Even when sedation or analgesia is administered, the child may have periods of **wakefulness** or **pain**. There currently is *no* proven assessment to determine pain and anxiety in the child receiving neuromuscular blocking agents.

Adverse responses include apnea, disuse atrophy, prolonged neuromuscular blockade, and pressure ulcers. Nursing interventions should be used to reduce these adverse responses.

The child may have unrecognized periods of wakefulness. It is important to speak to the child to tell him or her what is happening. For example, if the child needs to be suctioned, he or she should be informed that this will be done. If an alarm is going off, the child may be scared and require assurance that he or she is safe.

The family needs to be included in the child's care. Because the child looks as if he or she is sleeping, the family needs to know that the child may be able to hear them. The family should be allowed to participate in the child's care as the level of illness allows.

9. What signs indicate that a child may be experiencing wakefulness or pain while on a neuromuscular blocking agent?

Alterations in vital signs
Pupillary changes
Tearing

10. How can the family participate in care while their child is receiving a neuromuscular blocking agent?

Family members can help by:

Applying lotions	Reading to the child
Performing passive range of motion	Playing music
Bathing the child	Updating the child on the family life
Seeing to oral care	

RESPIRATORY SYSTEM

11. What is noninvasive positive-pressure ventilation?

This is a mode of ventilatory support. Positive pressure is delivered via a full facemask, nasal mask, nasal prongs, or nasal pillows. There must be an adequate seal to deliver the desired pressure. In this form of ventilation, no endotracheal tube is passed through the vocal cords. Noninvasive ventilation can help minimize airway trauma and edema and minimize sedation and analgesia requirements, but it cannot achieve the same level of ventilation as **endotracheal intubation** and **mechanical ventilation**.

12. When is noninvasive positive-pressure ventilation indicated?

- To help maintain upper airway patency
- To augment spontaneous respiration
- To increase functional residual capacity
- To prevent atelectasis
- To decrease work of breathing

13. On a machine providing noninvasive ventilation, what do the terms *IPAP* and *EPAP* indicate?

IPAP is **inspiratory positive airway pressure**, or the amount of pressure being delivered to the airways on inspiration. This is prescribed in centimeters (cm) of H_2O (range, 6–20 cm H_2O). IPAP augments the patient's spontaneous breath. IPAP is initiated when the machine senses that the patient has begun to inspire and terminates when the machine senses that the patient in no longer in the inspiratory phase of ventilation.

EPAP is **expiratory positive airway pressure**, or the pressure delivered to the patient at the end of expiration and in between breaths. EPAP helps maintain the patient's functional residual capacity and prevents atelectasis. The general range for EPAP is 3–8 cm H_2O. In some clinical situations, EPAP is used alone without IPAP.

14. What specific conditions must be monitored when caring for a patient on noninvasive ventilation?
- **Skin breakdown** resulting from snug fit and constant pressure of the mask or prongs being used to deliver the noninvasive ventilation
- **Eye and nasal irritation** or dryness resulting from high flow gas in these areas
- **Abdominal distention** resulting from positive pressure escaping into the abdomen

15. How can skin breakdown be prevented?

A skin barrier film should be placed between the mask and the skin to promote skin protection. The mask should be removed for short breaks during the day to clean the mask, assess the skin, and increase blood flow to the area.

16. Identify indications that noninvasive ventilation is failing and endotracheal intubation is necessary.

Hemodynamic instability
Worsening oxygenation
Difficulty in clearing secretions
Increase in agitation or confusion, altered mentation
Loss of ability to cough or gag

17. Differentiate between respiratory distress and respiratory failure.

Respiratory distress is the child's efforts to increase minute ventilation to compensate for impaired gas exchange. Quantifying respiratory distress is subjective and open to evaluator interpretation of symptoms. Typically a child with respiratory distress shows tachypnea, difficulty speaking, grunting, nasal flaring, tracheal tugging, retractions of the muscles of breathing, anxiety, and tachycardia. **Respiratory failure** is failure of compensatory mechanisms to meet oxygenation and ventilation demands of the body. Typically a child with respiratory failure shows depressed respiratory effort and respiratory rate, apnea, bradycardia, depressed level of consciousness, and cyanosis.

A child who previously was irritable with increased work of breathing and respiratory distress who now is sleeping with a lower respiratory rate and decreased work of breathing possibly is progressing to respiratory failure and requires prompt intervention.

18. On assessment of a newly admitted child with respiratory syncytial virus bronchiolitis, you notice the child is not breathing. What should you do?

For an **unwitnessed respiratory arrest**, the first action is to determine unresponsiveness and call for help. Next, open the airway and assess for breathing. If the child is not breathing, initiate bag-valve-mask ventilation. Assess for chest rise and fall. After giving two breaths, assess for a pulse. If the child has a pulse, continue to provide artificial breathing until a stable airway can be placed. For a **witnessed respiratory arrest**, open the airway and provide bag-valve-mask ventilation until a stable airway can be placed. For a complete algorithm for respiratory arrest management, see the American Heart Association's *Pediatric Advanced Life Support*.

19. How is the appropriate size endotracheal tube determined for a child?

By the size of the child's small finger or by the following equation:

$$\frac{16 + \text{age (years)}}{4}$$

In children with **congenital anomalies**, a half-size smaller endotracheal tube usually is appropriate.

20. Give examples of appropriate tube sizes based on a child's age.

AGE	ENDOTRACHEAL TUBE SIZE
Premature infant	2.5–3.0
Newborn	3.0
Newborn to 6 mo	3.5
6–12 mo	3.5–4.0
1–2 yr	4.0–4.5
3–4 yr	4.5–5.0
5–6 yr	5.0–5.5
7–8 yr	5.5–6.0
9–10 yr	6.0–6.5
11–12 yr	6.5–7.0
≥ 13 yr	7.0–7.5

21. How can the nurse determine if the endotracheal tube is in the trachea?
- Listen for presence of bilateral lung sounds.
- Evaluate for the presence of condensation in the endotracheal tube.
- Measure the presence of exhaled carbon dioxide with a disposable or end-tidal carbon dioxide detector.
- Identify the presence of the endotracheal tube on a chest radiograph.
- Have direct laryngoscopy performed by a clinician skilled in this procedure.

22. Identify complications of endotracheal intubation.
Complications of the intubation procedure

Soft tissue laceration or hematoma	Right main stem intubation
Dental damage	Esophageal intubation
Aspiration of gastric contents	Cardiac dysrhythmias resulting from hypoxia

Complications during intubation
Accidental extubation
Obstruction of the endotracheal tube (secretions, kinking, biting)
Increased resistance to breathing
Long-term sequelae of intubation

Laryngeal, tracheal, or vocal cord tissue damage or edema	Pressure sores of the soft tissues
	Subcutaneous emphysema
Infection	Subglottic stenosis

23. List complications of nasotracheal intubation.
- Epistaxis
- Trauma to the adenoids
- Obstruction of the eustachian tube leading to otitis media, sinusitis, and pressure necrosis of the nares

24. List the benefits of nasotracheal intubation.
- Improved patient comfort
- Decreased disturbance from oral secretions
- Easy to secure
- Decreased risk for dislodgment
- Elimination of tube obstruction as a result of biting
- Facilitation of oral care

25. What do you do when a tracheostomy placed less than 1 week prior becomes dislodged?

Within the first week of tracheostomy insertion, the tract has not yet had a chance to epithelialize, so inadvertent dislodgment is an **emergency situation**. The child should be positioned with the neck extended. The stay sutures that are placed when the initial tracheostomy is placed are sutured to the inside of the trachea. These sutures must be pulled gently upward and away from midline to reexpose the stoma. In a spontaneously breathing patient, if neither a new tracheostomy tube nor an endotracheal tube can be passed, an oxygen catheter should be inserted through the stoma to provide oxygen until the otolaryngologist can replace the tracheostomy tube. If assisted ventilation is required, the stoma site can be covered with gauze, and the patient can be bag mask ventilated or intubated in the usual fashion.

26. List the equipment required when performing a tracheostomy tube change in a patient with a well-established tracheotomy.
- Same size tracheostomy tube as patient currently has and one size smaller
- Suction
- Suction catheters
- Oxygen bag device
- Cardiorespiratory monitoring with pulse oximetry
- Gauze with soap and water, one dry gauze
- New set of tracheostomy tube ties or securing device
- Second person, if possible
- Lubricant

27. How is a well-established tracheotomy changed?

Two people are needed to for this task:

1. Person 1 opens the package, ensures the obturator is in place and can be removed easily from the tracheostomy tube, and then lightly lubricates the tracheostomy tube to be inserted.

2. If the patient is chronically ventilated, the second person should preoxygenate the patient.

3. Person 2 removes the current tracheostomy tube and assesses and cleans and dries the skin around the stoma site briefly while the tube is out.

4. Person 1 gently inserts the fresh tracheostomy tube and removes the obturator.

5. If the patient is chronically ventilated, person 2 should apply an oxygen bag to the patient.

6. The patient is assessed for comfort breathing, breath sounds, color, and saturation.

7. The new tracheostomy ties are secured.

8. The patient is assessed again for tolerance of the procedure.

9. The ventilator, oxygen, or humidity is replaced.

28. What must be done when a patient with a well-established tracheotomy develops tachypnea, respiratory distress, cyanosis, or decreased breath sounds?

It must be assumed that the **tracheostomy tube is obstructed** until proved otherwise. Obstruction is common as a result of secretions. The child should be ventilated with 100% oxygen and positioned with the head and neck extended to visualize the stoma site, and a suction catheter should be passed. If the suction catheter cannot pass through the tube, the tube is obstructed and must be removed and a new tube placed. After the new tube is placed, the patient should be reassessed for airway patency, breathing, and color.

29. How should the nurse approach blood gas analysis?
Two basic aspects of breathing are assessed: **ventilation and oxygenation** and **acid-base balance**.

Blood Gases (Uncompensated Values)

	pH	CO_2	BICARBONATE
Normal	7.35–7.45	35–45	22–26
Respiratory acidosis	< 7.35	> 45	Normal
Respiratory alkalosis	> 7.45	< 45	Normal
Metabolic acidosis	< 7.35	Normal	< 22
Metabolic alkalosis	> 7.45	Normal	≥ 26

Oxygenation is evaluated with the Pao_2 value on the blood gas; a value < 80 mmHg represents **hypoxemia** (this may be normal for a child with congenital heart disease).

30. Name the three primary pathologic factors causing airflow obstruction in children with asthma.
1. Bronchial muscle spasm
2. Mucosal edema
3. Mucus plugging

31. Explain the pathologic process of airflow obstruction in children with asthma.
Airflow obstruction on inspiration and expiration leads to an **overinflation** of the lungs. **Ventilation-perfusion mismatching** occurs because neither airflow obstruction nor perfusion is universally disturbed. This process causes a significant increase in physiologic dead space in overinflated areas of the lungs and a shuntlike effect in underinflated areas.

32. What kind of breath sound is most alarming when assessing a child with asthma?
Absent breath sounds. No breath sounds require immediate intervention. This is a sign that the airflow obstruction has become so severe that no ventilation is occurring at all.

33. What is heliox?
A mixture of **helium** and **oxygen**, usually 30% oxygen mixed with 70% helium or 40% oxygen mixed with 60% helium.

34. How does heliox improve airway obstruction?
Helium is seven times less dense than nitrogen. Thus, the heliox mixture is a much lighter gas than nitrogen and oxygen. This promotes laminar flow of gas, decreasing turbulent flow of gas and increasing gas delivery around areas of obstruction. Heliox can facilitate the delivery of inhaled medications, such as **albuterol**, to the lower airways.

35. In caring for a patient with status asthmaticus, how long until the intravenous steroid that was administered begins to take effect?
It takes steroids approximately 4–6 hours until their effects are seen. Patients may require more aggressive management until the steroids take effect, then may improve several hours after the dose is given.

36. How do intravenous steroids help?
Steroids help decrease the inflammation in the airways.

37. What is a pulsus paradoxus?
An accentuation of the usual decrease in systemic blood pressure on inspiration.

38. How can pulsus paradoxus be detected?

Pulsus paradoxus can be appreciated on **physical examination** by a decrease in amplitude in the palpated pulse during inspiration. When auscultating the blood pressure, the Korotkoff sounds are present only on expiration. It can be noted on the **monitor** of a patient with an **arterial line**. A significant pulsus paradoxus is a measurable fall in pulse pressure on inspiration of ≥ 12 mmHg. This reflects the reduction in blood flow returning to the left side of the heart.

39. In what conditions can pulsus paradoxus be seen?

Cardiac tamponade   Hypovolemia
Status asthmaticus   Constrictive pericarditis
Tension pneumothorax   Restrictive cardiomyopathy

40. What is acute respiratory distress syndrome (ARDS)?

ARDS is an illness characterized by acute onset of respiratory symptoms, bilateral infiltrates on chest radiograph, and no evidence of left atrial hypertension as a causative factor for the prior symptoms. ARDS is associated with a constellation of clinical, radiologic, and physiologic abnormalities.

41. Which illness most commonly precedes ARDS?

Sepsis.

42. What other conditions typically precede ARDS?

Trauma   Shock
Pulmonary aspiration   Multiple transfusions
Pneumonia   Near-drowning
Airway disease   After bone marrow transplant

43. How is ARDS treated?

The treatment of ARDS is supportive. There currently is no curative therapy. Management includes oxygen therapy, positive end-expiratory pressure, limiting peak inspiratory pressure, maximizing oxygen delivery, minimizing oxygen consumption, maintaining fluid balance, nutritional support, and therapies aimed at treating the preceding disease process. **High-frequency oscillatory ventilation** may be used if conventional (standard) ventilation fails to support the child with ARDS. **Extracorporeal membrane oxygenation** may be used if conventional or high-frequency oscillatory ventilation no longer is providing adequate therapy.

44. What therapies are currently being researched in the supportive care of ARDS?

Prone positioning
Surfactant replacement
Inhaled nitric oxide

45. What are the key elements of nursing care for the child with ARDS?

• Ensure patency of the artificial airway.
• Assess respiratory system frequently and monitor for changes.
• Maintain and monitor ventilatory parameters.
• Assess synchrony with the ventilator.
• Maintain and monitor oxygen delivery system.
• Monitor oxygenation.
• Monitor ventilation.
• Maintain alarm systems.
• Monitor vital signs routinely.
• Assess perfusion.
• Monitor intake and output.
• Maintain comfort.

• Maintain appropriate positioning.
• Provide routine range of motion (as tolerated) if patient is immobile.

46. What is IMV/SIMV ventilation mode?

Intermittent mandatory ventilation (IMV) is a mode of ventilation with a set respiratory rate delivered to the child. It also supports the child when he or she takes breaths in addition to the set respiratory rate. **Synchronized intermittent mandatory ventilation (SIMV)** is the same as IMV except it delivers the set respiratory rate in synchrony with the child's own breaths.

47. Explain volume control ventilation.

Volume ventilation is a mode in which the volume of each breath is set on the ventilator. A child may be receiving SIMV in volume control mode with a set respiratory rate of 12 breaths/min and a tidal volume of 100 mL. This means that with each of the 12 breaths, the child has 100 mL of gas delivered to the lungs. The pressure required to deliver each 100-mL breath may vary. If the child has stiff lungs, it will take more pressure to deliver the set volume. Conversely, if the child has compliant lungs, the pressure needed to deliver the volume will be lower.

48. Explain pressure control ventilation.

Pressure ventilation is a mode in which the pressure of each breath is set on the ventilator. The child on SIMV in pressure control mode with a set respiratory rate of 12 breaths/min and pressure control of 20 has each of the 12 breaths delivered until the pressure reaches 20. The volume of each breath may vary for the pressure delivered. If the child has stiff lungs, the volume delivered to reach the set pressure will be low. If the child has compliant lungs, the volume to reach the set pressure will be higher.

49. Explain pressure support ventilation.

Pressure support ventilation can be used in addition to volume control and pressure control or independently as a weaning mode. In the pressure support mode alone, there is a set pressure on the ventilator without a mandatory respiratory rate. The child initiates his or her own breath that is sensed by the ventilator, and the ventilator delivers a pressure to support the breath to the child. Each breath reaches the set pressure and, similar to pressure control, could have a variable volume.

50. Explain volume support ventilation.

Volume support ventilation is similar to pressure support except that the volume is set without a set respiratory rate, and the pressure could vary with each breath.

51. What is the difference between the pressure support/volume support and pressure control/volume control modes?

With pressure control/volume control, there is a set respiratory rate, and with pressure support/volume support, there may or may not be a set respiratory rate.

52. What key elements of nursing care are important for the child who is intubated and ventilated?

Nursing care is the same as for the child with ARDS (see question 45).

CARDIOVASCULAR SYSTEM

53. Which congenital cardiac anomalies are acyanotic defects?

Atrial septal defect	Aortic stenosis
Ventricular septal defect	Pulmonary stenosis
Patent ductus arteriosus	Atrioventricular septal defect
Coarctation of the aorta	

54. Which congenital cardiac anomalies are cyanotic defects?

Transposition of the great arteries   Truncus arteriosus
Tricuspid atresia   Hypoplastic left heart syndrome
Tetralogy of Fallot   Single ventricle
Pulmonary atresia with intact ventricular septum   Double-outlet right ventricle
Total anomalous pulmonary venous connection   Double-inlet left ventricle

55. What are some of the complications after cardiac surgery?

Inadequate tissue perfusion   Pulmonary hypertension
Inadequate intravascular volume   Increased systemic afterload
Rhythm disturbances   Myocardial dysfunction
Tamponade

56. Differentiate between cardioversion and defibrillation.

	CARDIOVERSION	DEFIBRILLATION
Definition	Synchronized release energy timed with the R wave of the ECG	Asynchronous delivery of energy to critical mass of myocardial cells
Indications	Tachyarrhythmia with cardiovascular compromise	Ventricular fibrillation or pulseless ventricular tachycardia
Dosage	0.5 J/kg May increase to 1 J/kg if rhythm persists	2 J/kg May increase to 4 J/kg if rhythm persists
Special considerations	*Synchronized* button must be turned on. Patient must be attached to ECG for synchrony to occur Must press and hold discharge button and wait for countershock to occur	First dose is 2 J/kg, then 4 J/kg and if a third dose is needed, 4 J/kg If rhythm returns, use same energy dose that terminated it Announce defibrillation ("All clear!") to avoid shocking others

57. How are drugs administered through an endotracheal tube?

Drugs should be diluted with 3–5 mL of saline, administered into the endotracheal tube, and bagged into the patient.

58. Which drugs can be administered through an endotracheal tube?

Atropine
Lidocaine
Epinephrine
Naloxone

59. What is adenosine?

A drug that slows conduction through the atrioventricular node, causing bradycardia and possibly asystole. **Adenosine** is indicated for the treatment of **supraventricular tachycardia**.

60. What is the dosage and administration of adenosine?

The initial dose is 0.1 mg/kg. The highest single dose should not exceed 12 mg or 0.3 mg/kg. The half-life of adenosine is 10 seconds, and the effective duration time is < 2 minutes. Because of this, adenosine must be administered rapidly and followed rapidly by 2–5 mL of saline.

61. What do the different settings mean on a temporary pacemaker?

FIRST LETTER	SECOND LETTER	THIRD LETTER
Chamber paced	Chamber sensed	Mode of response to sensed event
A = Atrium	A = Atrium	T = Triggered
V = Ventricle	V = Ventricle	I = Inhibited
D = Dual	D = Dual	D = Triggered and inhibited
	O = None	O = None

For example, a child with a DDD pacer has the atria and ventricles sensed and paced. The mode of response to a sensored event means that the pacer will allow time for a native electrical activity to occur, and if it does, the pacer will not provide a stimulus. If the native electrical activity does not occur, the pacer will provide the stimulus.

62. Define inotropy and chronotropy.

Inotropy is the influence of the muscle contraction. Inotropy can be negative, decreasing muscle contraction, or positive, increasing muscle contraction. **Chronotropy** is the influence of the rate of contractility of the muscle. These terms are generally used to describe the action of cardiac medications.

63. Describe the common cardiac support medications.

MEDICATION	ACTION	DOSAGE	SIDE EFFECTS
Dopamine	β-adrenergic → positive inotropy, chronotropy, vasodilation activity α-adrenergic as dose increases → inotropy and vasoconstriction activity	Generally, 2–5 µg/kg/min is used for renal vasodilatory effects and is controversial 2–20 µg/kg/min is the general range of therapeutic dosing	Tachycardia, increased myocardial workload, mild mismatch of myocardial oxygen demand and consumption. Dopamine extravasation → necrosis, gangrene
Dobutamine	Selective inotropy, limited chronotropy and vasoconstriction activity	2–20 µg/kg/min	Tachycardia, arrhythmias, expressive fluctuations in blood pressure, headache, anxiety, and tumors
Epinephrine	β-adrenergic → positive inotropy and chronotropy activity α-adrenergic as dose increases → positive inotropy, vasoconstriction activity	0.1–1 µg/kg/min	Central nervous system excitation, tachycardia, ventricular ectopy, tachyarrhythmias, severe angina, hypertension, mismatch of myocardial oxygen demand and consumption
Milrinone	Potent inotropy with systemic and pulmonary vasodilation activity	Loading dose 0.5–0.75 µg/kg over 20 minutes 0.5–1 µg/kg/min	Arrhythmias and hypotension

64. What types of shock are commonly seen in the critical care patient?

TYPE	AGE GROUP	CAUSATIVE FACTORS
Hypovolemic shock	Infant and toddler All ages: as a result of hemorrhagic trauma and burns	Usually results from fluid and electrolyte losses owing to vomiting and/or diarrhea. It also can be due to redistribution of blood volume (e.g., caused by increased capillary permeability as a result of bacterial toxins) in all age categories
Septic shock	All ages: common in patients with compromised immune systems (oncology or transplant patients)	Associated with an overwhelming infection and subsequent failure of the body to respond to the invasion of the organism
Cardiogenic shock	Most commonly seen in patients with arrhythmias or cardiomyopathy and-after cardiovascular surgery. May be secondary to sepsis or acid-base imbalances	Occurs as a result of the heart's impaired ability to pump blood and resultant decline in cardiac output

65. What are the stages of shock?

1. **Compensated.** The body's compensatory mechanisms are activated in response to the insult it has received. These mechanisms include activation of the sympathetic nervous system and release of aldosterone and antidiuretic hormone (ADH). Vital organ function is supported. It is difficult to differentiate this stage of shock because blood pressure may be normal. The nurse should look for tachycardia, tachypnea, cool and pale extremities, restlessness, and decreased urine output.

2. **Uncompensated or progressive.** Compensatory mechanisms fail to support the delivery of oxygen to the tissues; the body loses its ability to autoregulate the blood pressure, resulting in decreased cardiac output. The patient now appears cold and cyanotic, has weak peripheral pulses, is lethargic, is mottled, and has poor respiratory effort. Immediate interventions are necessary to prevent progression.

3. **Irreversible.** Evidence of **multisystem organ failure** is prevalent despite efforts at interventions. Total body failure and death ensue.

66. What are the general principles of treatment of shock in the critical care unit?

- Initial treatment follows the **ABC guidelines: airway, breathing, and circulation**. Oxygen should be the first medication delivered to the patient. The goal is to restore the delivery of adequate oxygen and nutrients to the tissue.
- **Vascular access** should be established according to the Pediatric Advanced Life Support guidelines.
- **Fluid resuscitation** should be started if indicated, with addition of medications to manipulate preload, myocardial contractility, heart rate, and afterload when there is an adequate circulating volume. The goal is enhancement of cardiac output and stabilization of systemic arterial blood pressure.
- Essential to treatment is **evaluation** of the interventions and constant **assessment and reassessment** of the patient to determine the effectiveness of the treatment.

67. What does the nurse need to know about monitoring the patient in shock?

Level of consciousness. It is key to note the subtle changes that may be present in a child. A child who does not seem to recognize his or her mother is likely oxygen deficient and needs immediate attention. A child who progresses from awake and alert to lethargic requires immediate attention.

Circulation. Assess peripheral circulation by looking at capillary refill, peripheral pulses, color, and temperature. Shock is a problem of decreased tissue perfusion, not decreased blood pressure. A child in compensated shock may have normal or slightly elevated blood pressure; decreased blood pressure indicates **decompensated shock**. A brisk capillary refill is < 2 seconds. Assess pulse for rate, rhythm, and quality. **Bradycardia** in shock is an ominous sign. Sometimes patients who are tachycardic or who have poor tissue perfusion are difficult to monitor for pulse oximeter readings.

Hydration. Urine output is an important indicator when assessing for shock. Adequate urine output is 1 mL/kg/h in children.

Breathing. Monitor respiratory rate and depth and work of breathing. Early in shock, hypoxia stimulates the patient to breathe deeper and faster.

Invasive monitoring. As shock progresses, the use of indwelling arterial catheters and central catheters allows for more information for treatment. The nurse must be diligent in maintaining these lines and calibrating the transducer for accurate readings.

68. How do you fluid resuscitate a child in hypovolemic shock?

The current standard is to use isotonic **crystalloids** (lactated Ringer's, 0.9% sodium chloride) for fluid resuscitation because they are more readily available and cost-effective. A bolus of 20 mL/kg is given first. After each bolus, the patient is assessed. Repeat boluses of 20 mL/kg are given until adequacy of systemic perfusion or evidence of systemic and pulmonary venous congestion and myocardial dysfunction is observed. If the patient is losing fluid through hemorrhage, he or she requires a transfusion of red blood cells to restore oxygen-carrying capacity. The total volume given to the patient may exceed the total volume lost because of expanded capacitance of the vascular space and dysfunction of the cellular membrane (capillary leak syndrome).

69. What about fluid resuscitation in a child with septic shock?

Volumes > 100–200 mL/kg may be given within the first 4 hours and are associated with improved outcomes. It is vital to assess the patient to prevent volume overload.

70. How does treatment of cardiogenic shock differ from treatment of other types of shock?

Because reduction of oxygen and substrate delivery to the tissues is due to abnormalities of cardiac rhythm or function in cardiogenic shock, treatment includes drugs designed to augment contractility or reduce elevated systemic vascular resistance or both. Efforts are made to maximize oxygen delivery and minimize oxygen demands. Preload augmentation by volume expansion must be used carefully in this case because the volume to be given depends on ventricular compliance. Attention should be given to the physical examination and the central venous pressure—a central venous pressure > 7–10 indicates myocardial dysfunction. Next, contractility needs to be optimized. A β_1 inotrope, such as **dobutamine**, is helpful in myocardial depression, and **milrinone** is used to improve diastolic function. Afterload also must be optimized in cardiogenic shock because the increased systemic vascular resistance can compromise myocardial function. The most common of these drugs are **nitroprusside** and **nitroglycerin**. Care must be taken to ensure adequate circulating volume because these drugs have the capability of producing hypotension in hypovolemia.

71. What are the phases of septic shock?

Septic shock is progressive in nature and occurs in three phases.

1. The first phase, **hyperdynamic shock**, reflects the compensated phase that results from tachycardia, increased ventricular end-diastolic volume, and a fall in systemic vascular resistance. There is a clinical state of systemic vasodilation and high cardiac output. The child may appear flushed, with warm extremities, bounding pulses, fever, and mild mental confusion. Tachypnea and respiratory alkalosis are present.

2. In the second phase, **hyperdynamic uncompensated shock**, a child presents with clinical decompensated shock: Extremities are cool, vascular resistance is high, and cardiac output is low. Metabolic acidosis, systemic and pulmonary edema, hypoxemia, tachypnea, and increased work of breathing are present.

3. The third phase, **hypodynamic** or **cardiogenic shock**, involves severe circulatory compromise with cold extremities, hypotension, severe acidosis, and multisystem organ failure.

72. What is the treatment for septic shock?

One of the goals of treatment is to eradicate the infection through antibiotics, although the causative agent may not be identified. Support of the **cardiorespiratory system** is crucial but complicated because of two primary categories of hemodynamic instability: (1) hypovolemia associated with severe capillary leak and inadequate volume resuscitation and (2) intrinsic cardiac pump failure. Septic shock is a combination of hypovolemic and cardiogenic shocks. Early aggressive **fluid resuscitation** has been proven to improve outcomes.

73. Which drugs are used for pediatric septic shock?

Of the agents available to improve cardiac output, **dopamine** and **epinephrine** have been chosen at various pediatric institutions as the first-line drugs of choice. **Epinephrine** can provide β-adrenergic support of myocardial contractility and peripheral vascular effects. **Dopamine** has β-adrenergic effects on the myocardium, α-adrenergic effects on the peripheral vasculature, and dopaminergic effects on the renal and splanchnic vasculature.

74. What are the complications of septic shock?

ARDS may develop, necessitating the use of high-frequency ventilation or extracorporeal membrane oxygenation.

Disseminated intravascular coagulopathy (DIC) may develop. The nurse needs to be prepared to facilitate the administration of multiple blood products and frequent laboratory draws to keep the patient in a steady-state.

Multisystem organ failure may develop and is associated with high morbidity and mortality rates.

FLUID MANAGEMENT

75. Describe the 4, 2, 1 method for calculating maintenance intravenous fluids for an infant or child with normal renal function and cardiac status.
  - First 10 kg: 4 mL/kg up to 10 kg.
  - Second 10 kg: 40 mL (from the first 10 kg), plus 2 mL/kg for second 10 kg.
  - Third 10 kg and above: 60 mL (from first 20 kg), plus 1 mL/kg above 20 kg.
    Generally, patients weighing > 60 kg receive 100 mL/hr.
    Example: A 22-kg child would receive:
    First 10 kg: 4 mL/kg × 10 kg = 40 mL
    Second 10 kg: 2 mL/kg × 10 kg = 20 mL
    Last 2 kg: 1 mL/kg × 2 kg = 2 mL
    40 mL + 20 mL + 2 mL = 62 mL/hr for maintenance IV fluids.

ONCOLOGY, HEMATOLOGY, AND INFECTIOUS DISEASE

76. Under what conditions is an oncology patient admitted to the critical care unit?

Children with oncologic disease are admitted to the critical care unit for complications resulting from the **malignant tumor** or **disease** or from the effects of **antineoplastic therapy**.

77. **List types of patients who are seen in this setting.**
   - Children with a new diagnosis who have a life-threatening complication of the tumor or disease (e.g., a newly diagnosed child with acute lymphoblastic leukemia with a white blood cell count of 300,000)
   - Children who require intense monitoring and close observation during or after a high-risk procedure (e.g., an exchange transfusion)
   - Children with major complications resulting from ongoing disease or consequences of therapy (most critical care admissions are children who are **neutropenic** and become **septic**)

78. **A patient has just been admitted from the oncology floor, and the family appears guarded. What can the nurse do to help the family?**
   Families of children with oncologic disease have special psychosocial and medical needs. They are dealing with the traumatic events of the child's illness and now are in a new environment. Many have been on the oncology floor for several admissions, and they are familiar and comfortable with the staff and plan of care. The pediatric intensive care unit nurse can facilitate the transition by carefully explaining routines, listening when the parents express their needs and fears, and designating a primary care nurse for that child whom the family can see on a daily basis and with whom they can become comfortable. The nurse can facilitate communication between the oncology team and the critical care team so that the family gets accurate and consistent communication and both teams can develop consistent goals. Care conferences with all members of the team and the parents help this process.

79. **What is hyperleukocytosis?**
   A peripheral white blood cell count > 100,000/mm^3, more likely to occur in children with acute nonlymphocytic leukemia and acute myelogenous leukemia. Critical values of 300,000/mm^3 have been associated with central nervous system or pulmonary complications.

80. **What central nervous system and pulmonary complications are associated with hyperleukocytosis?**

Central nervous system		Pulmonary
Blurred vision	Delirium	Dyspnea
Confusion	Stupor	Hypoxemia
Agitation	Intracranial hemorrhage	Acidosis

81. **How is hyperleukocytosis treated in the critical care unit?**
   - Fluids are administered to reduce blood viscosity.
   - Transfusions usually are not given unless the child's hemoglobin is critically low. If a transfusion is given, care should be taken not to raise the child's hemoglobin levels to > 10 g/dL.
   - Diuretics should be discouraged because resultant diuresis increases the viscosity of the blood.
   - When white blood cell count is > 300,000/mm^3, **exchange transfusion** may be indicated to reduce blood viscosity.
   - Another approach is **leukopheresis**, although a disadvantage with this treatment is the necessity of anticoagulation therapy and occasional vascular access problem.
   - Critical care also includes support of ventilation and oxygenation, especially in children with white blood cell counts > 300,000/mm^3; it is necessary to monitor closely for any signs and symptoms of **intracranial hemorrhage** (often there is a complaint of a unilateral headache).

82. **Describe the complications of bone marrow transplant.**
   1. Most bone marrow transplant patients admitted to the critical care unit exhibit signs and symptoms of **infection**, the leading cause of morbidity and mortality in this population. A

pulmonary infection that requires intubation to support oxygenation and ventilation presents a greater risk of morbidity and mortality.

2. **Acute graft-versus-host disease** can occur and presents an even higher risk for infection because of the loss of skin integrity. Any blood products transfused to the patient should be irradiated to prevent the transfusion of active T lymphocytes from product donors.

3. The development of **veno-occlusive disease** is possible typically 1-3 weeks post-transplant. Fibrous deposits block small venules of the liver so that there is obstructed flow from the liver, resulting in ascites.

83. What is disseminated intravascular coagulopathy (DIC)?

A syndrome associated with the rapid consumption of clotting proteins and platelets because of the excessive production of **thrombin** and **activated factor X**. Fibrinogen is converted into fibrin, the major component of normal clots, and microthrombi are deposited throughout the vascular bed. **Fibrin deposits** attract and trap platelets and red blood cells and consume clotting factors. As the process continues, **fibrin split products** are produced and, if not cleared, enhance anticoagulation. An increase in the fibrin split products is the cardinal sign of DIC.

84. Name causes of DIC.

Infection (most common cause)
Massive trauma with shock
Malignancies
Immune diseases

85. List laboratory findings consistent with DIC.

Increased prothrombin time
Increased partial thromboplastin time
Increased fibrin split products
Decreased fibrinogen
Decreased platelets

86. How is DIC treated?

- Replacement of blood products (platelets, fresh-frozen plasma, and cryoprecipitate) and control and prevention of any further bleeding are most important.
- Recognition and treatment of the precipitating cause is essential (because infection is the most common cause, identification and eradication of the infiltrating organism is key).

87. How many milliliters of blood make up a child's total blood volume?

Children < 1 year old: 75–80 mL/kg
Children > 1 year old: 70 mL/kg

88. When performing an exchange blood transfusion, which metabolic derangements must be monitored for closely?

Hyperkalemia, **hypocalcemia**, and **hypomagnesemia** are the major metabolic derangements that can occur during exchange transfusions. Packed red blood cells are stored at a temperature of 4°C to increase their shelf life and to decrease their metabolic demands. Blood undergoes significant alterations during storage, and the longer the blood is stored, the more likely there are alterations. Even with improvements in blood preservation, 1% of cells may undergo osmotic lysis during storage as a result of failure of the sodium-potassium adenosine triphosphatase–dependent pump. The lysed cells release free hemoglobin and potassium, and a high plasma concentration of potassium is in transfused blood, resulting in **hyperkalemia**. Preservatives used to store blood contain citrates. Tissues, particularly the liver, must metabolize the citrate. Before the citrate is eliminated, it may bind covalent cations, such as calcium and magnesium, resulting in **hypocalcemia** and **hypomagnesemia**. Documented hypocalcemia and hypomagnesemia must be treated.

89. Why do the cells in sickle cell disease cause complications such as pain crisis, priapism, and acute chest syndrome?

The complications ultimately are due to the **sickling** of red blood cells. This leads to vascular occlusion and inability to deliver oxygen to target organs. There also is distortion of cell morphology, changes in cellular viscosity, and vascular sludging, which can result in organ infarction. Patients who are acidotic, febrile, dehydrated, or hypoxic are more likely to develop manifestations of vaso-occlusive disease.

90. Why does transfusion therapy help patients in sickle cell crisis?

In most circumstances, patients with sickle cell disease do not require red blood cell transfusion to treat the anemia. Patients are given transfusions to reduce the number of circulating sickled cells. This helps reduce or prevent complications from the existing sickled cells. The goal is to increase hematocrit and decrease the hemoglobin S (sickle) concentration. It is important to screen the donated blood for sickle cell disease.

91. Name common reasons for hospital admission in children with sickle cell disease.

Acute chest syndrome, pain crisis, and priapism.

92. What are the symptoms of acute chest syndrome?

Tachypnea	Cough
Chest pain	Drop in baseline hemoglobin
Oxygen requirement	Infiltrate on chest radiograph
Fever	

93. Identify the routes of entry of organisms that cause meningitis.

- Hematogenous (directly from the blood)
- Direct extension into meninges (may result from an infection of the paranasal sinuses and mastoid region)
- Direct penetration (i.e., trauma)

94. In which clinical situations is a lumbar puncture (LP) potentially hazardous to the patient?

- Hemodynamic instability precluding appropriate patient positioning
- Increased ICP
- Presence of a brain abscess or mass

95. What is an alternative method to obtain spinal fluid if LP is too hazardous?

Ventricular puncture (performed by skilled personnel).

96. Can patients be treated without obtaining a cerebrospinal fluid sample?

Yes. These children may be treated with appropriate antibiotic coverage.

97. Describe the correct position for an infant or child undergoing lumbar puncture.

The patient should be placed on the edge of the bed or examination table toward the practitioner performing the procedure. The patient should have the neck flexed and knees brought up to a fetal position. The shoulders should be perpendicular to the bed. The child should be held securely, with attention to the fact that **cardiorespiratory arrest** can occur if the child is held too firmly owing to obstruction of the airway or impedance of venous return. Cardiorespiratory monitoring is essential.

Alternate positioning for an infant undergoing lumbar puncture is to hold the patient sitting up, flexing the knees up to the abdomen.

HEAD INJURY/NEUROLOGY

98. A child just was admitted to the pediatric intensive care unit after being involved in a motor vehicle crash. How can the nurse rapidly assess the child's level of consciousness?

The easiest assessment tool is the **Glasgow Coma Scale**. This scale evaluates the child in three areas: **eye opening**, **verbal response**, and **motor response**. Each area is scored individually, with the best response having the highest score. The Glasgow Coma Scale score can range from 3 to 15. Patients with a Glasgow Coma Scale score of ≤ 8 require intubation. This scale typically is used reliably for preschool children and older patients. A modified scale can be used for infants, which evaluates the infant in the same three areas with developmentally appropriate responses.

Glasgow Coma Scale

VARIABLE	PATIENT RESPONSE	SCORE
Eye opening	Spontaneous	4
	To voice	3
	To pain	2
	None	1
Verbal response	Oriented	5
	Confused	4
	Inappropriate	3
	Incomprehensible	2
	None	1
Motor response	Obeys verbal commands	6
	Localizes (to pain)	5
	Withdraws (to pain)	4
	Flexion (to pain, decorticate)	3
	Extension (to pain, decerebrate)	2
	None	1

99. Identify initial stabilization therapies for a child admitted after a motor vehicle crash.

1. Initial stabilization of the patient with a head injury starts with the **ABCs**.

2. A child with a head injury must be presumed to have a cervical spinal injury, so the **cervical spine** must be protected during intubation.

3. When the airway and ventilation are established, attention must be paid to establishing and maintaining **hemodynamic stability**.

4. **Hypotension** is common after head injury and may indicate blood loss, possibly from associated systemic injuries or inadequate vascular volume.

5. It is crucial to establish adequate cardiac output quickly and prevent secondary brain injury.

100. Define primary and secondary brain injury.

Primary brain injury occurs immediately after the trauma and may result in cell damage or death. **Secondary brain injury** is a result of the brain's response to the trauma, is a progressive process, and generally peaks in 3–5 days. Although prevention of the primary trauma may not be possible, prompt recognition and minimization of secondary injury can influence a child's outcome significantly.

101. Identify elements of secondary brain injury.

• Development of cerebral edema
• Loss of cerebral autoregulation
• Breakdown of the blood-brain barrier

102. What is the significance of clear fluid oozing from a child's ear?

This may indicate the presence of a **cerebrospinal fluid leak**. The fluid should be tested for the presence of glucose; if positive, the presence of cerebrospinal fluid should be considered.

103. When is ICP monitoring indicated?
- Patients with head injuries who are intubated and ventilated or in shock
- Patients with a Glasgow Coma Scale score of ≤ 6
- Patients with multiple contusions or compressed cisterns on computed tomography scan

104. How is ICP monitoring accomplished?

ICP monitoring devices can be inserted in the pediatric intensive care unit or in the operating room. These include:
- **Intraventricular devices**, which have the capability of monitoring and draining fluid
- **Intraparenchymal devices**, using a small fiber-optic catheter
- **Epidural monitors**, which have the advantage of ease of placement but have not been found to correlate well with the ventricular pressures

105. Why is ICP monitoring done?
- To intervene in the development of cerebral edema and prevent herniation
- To preserve the cerebral perfusion pressure (CPP)

106. How is CPP calculated?

The CPP is the difference between the mean arterial pressure (MAP) and the mean ICP:

$$CPP = MAP - ICP$$

107. What is a normal CPP value?

Normal CPP in children has not been determined, but as a general rule of thumb, a CPP of ≥ **50** is thought to maintain adequate cerebral blood flow.

108. Identify interventions to maintain CPP.
- Augmentation of the mean arterial pressure using vasopressors
- Various methods to decrease the ICP

109. When should the ICP be decreased?

Generally, when the ICP reaches 20 mmHg, measures should be taken to reduce the ICP, thereby increasing CPP.

110. What can be done to decrease the ICP?

1. **Hyperosmolar therapy.** Osmotic agents are used to shift free water from the interstitial and cellular space to the intravascular space, removing the interstitial water from the brain. The most common agent is **mannitol** (initial dose range, 0.5–1 g/kg). Serum electrolytes and osmolality must be monitored closely. When serum osmolality is > 310–320 mOsm/L, other therapies should be considered. A combination of mannitol and a loop diuretic, such as **furosemide**, also may be used. Fluid and electrolyte balances must be monitored to decrease the risk of neurologic sequelae resulting from abnormalities.

2. **Cerebrospinal fluid drainage.** Drainage of cerebrospinal fluid from a ventricular drain can reduce ICP. This is done continuously, maintaining a static ICP, or intermittently as a treatment for spikes of ICP. **Overdrainage** can end in ventricular collapse and loss of further ability to monitor.

3. **Barbiturates** decrease cerebral metabolism. Although barbiturate coma is effective in lowering the ICP, it carries the risk of hypotension and decreased cardiac output, risking integrity of the CPP. **Thiopental** is used to achieve rapid reduction of ICP prophylactically in situations in which the ICP is likely to rise (i.e., before suctioning).

4. **Neuromuscular blocking agents** reduce metabolic demand and therefore potentially decrease ICP. Analgesia and sedation must be used concurrently with neuromuscular blockade and serve to decrease ICP.

5. **Hyperventilation.** Hyperventilation previously was used to maintain a relative **hypocarbia** to reduce cerebral blood volume and ICP; however, the ICP also may rise in the presence of hypoxemia, so hyperventilation is reserved for situations when herniation is imminent.

111. What is status epilepticus?

A condition characterized by the repetition of epileptic seizures at brief intervals without recovery or consciousness between the attacks or by prolongation of a seizure as to realize a fixed and lasting condition (generally > 30 minutes). Critical care monitoring is necessary, especially after this time lapse because compensatory mechanisms of the body are failing, producing hypotension and shock, and the efforts to terminate the seizures create side effects, such as respiratory depression or apnea.

112. What are the nursing priorities when stabilizing a patient in status epilepticus?

1. Stabilization of the patient begins with the **ABCs**.

2. **Intubation** may be necessary if the patient already has been given drugs that have caused respiratory depression or if the patient remains hypoxic despite oxygen delivery. Because seizure activity needs to stop for intubation, **paralytic agents** are used. Paralytic agents do not effectively stop the seizure activity, just the movement. After intubation, the patient must be placed on a **ventilator**.

3. Attention must be given to maintain adequate **cardiac output** using fluids and vasopressors because hypotension or bradycardia or both may occur with prolonged seizures.

4. Although **hypoglycemia** is a rare cause of status epilepticus, it may complicate treatment, so determination of glucose and treatment of hypoglycemia is necessary.

113. What drugs are used for initial treatment of status epilepticus?

A combination of agents is used.

1. The **benzodiazepines** are used as a first-line drug because of their rapid onset. **Diazepam** (which has an onset of action of 1–2 minutes), **lorazepam** (which is preferred because of its longer duration of action), and **midazolam** (which not only has a quick onset of action, but also can be given intranasally), all have been used.

2. A longer acting agent, such as **phenytoin**, is then used. A loading dose of 20 mg/kg is given intravenously. Important considerations for use of intravenous phenytoin include compatibility. It precipitates in many fluids and should be given with a saline flush before and after. The rate of infusion is important: Phenytoin should be given slowly, not more than 0.5 mg/kg/min with a maximum of 50 mg/min. Infusions given too fast depress myocardial function and cause arrhythmias or cardiac standstill. All patients receiving intravenous phenytoin need to be on a cardiac monitor. **Fosphenytoin**, which metabolizes to phenytoin when given, has fewer side effects and toxicities but is more expensive. Its dose is expressed in phenytoin equivalents.

3. **Phenobarbital** is another long-lasting agent and is given if seizures are refractory to diazepam and phenytoin, although it frequently is used as the first-line agent. It has the slowest onset of action. Respiratory depression and hypotension are significant side effects of phenobarbital.

114. What can be done if the child is still having seizures?

Barbiturate coma should be considered. Advantages of this treatment are reduction of neuronal metabolic rate and ICP and the need for oxygen. Intubation and vascular access are imperative. Volume expanders and vasopressor infusions should be at the bedside. Because clinical seizure activity may not be seen, frequent, if not continuous, monitoring and interpretation of the **electroencephalogram** is essential to determine effectiveness of treatment. The disadvantage of this therapy is the hemodynamic instability that occurs as a result of the medications.

115. What agents are used to treat barbiturate coma?
- Thiopental infusions (frequently preferred because it has a shorter half-life and is eliminated quickly from the body)
- Pentobarbital infusions
- Intermittent doses of phenobarbital given at 20-minute intervals until burst suppression is achieved (there is no maximal dose, and levels of 340 µg/mL [therapeutic range is 15–40 µg/mL] have been necessary to achieve burst suppression)

METABOLISM/ENDOCRINOLOGY

116. What is diabetic ketoacidosis (DKA)?
DKA is a result of lack of insulin and resultant hyperglycemia, which can result in dehydration from osmotic diuresis. Acidosis is primarily the result of accumulation of ketoacids, but also can include lactic acidosis from hypoperfused tissues. A variety of electrolyte imbalances ensue.

117. Describe the presentation of DKA.
Many patients present with **low serum sodium** from loss in the urine, and **potassium** levels likewise are decreased. Potassium levels initially may be elevated as a result of the movement of potassium to the extracellular-intravascular compartment in exchange for hydrogen ions moving into the cell in acidosis. As a compensatory mechanism in response to metabolic acidosis, the patient develops **Kussmaul breathing** (deep, rapid respirations), which results in an increase in carbon dioxide exhalation and a fall in intravascular bicarbonate ion concentration.

118. What laboratory values indicate DKA?
Serum glucose > 300 mg/dL
Serum pH < 7.3
Serum bicarbonate < 15 mEq/L

119. When does a child with DKA need admission to the critical care unit?
A child may not need intensive care if there is a clear sensorium and good peripheral circulation present. In general, any newly diagnosed diabetic with moderate dehydration and acidosis or a known diabetic with significant acidosis and dehydration needs critical care. Patients who are younger than 2 years of age, have a pH < 7.0, or have altered mentation should be admitted to the critical care unit for close observation and treatment.

120. What fluids should be administered to patients with DKA?
Dehydration in DKA often is underestimated because of the shift of water from the intracellular to the extracellular compartment owing to **osmosis**. The goals of fluid administration are to replace the estimated deficit plus ongoing losses and give maintenance therapy. An initial fluid bolus of 10–20 mL/kg of normal saline is initially given over 1–2 hours. If the systemic perfusion is still not adequate, a second bolus may be necessary. The remainder of the fluid deficit is replaced over 24–48 hours to prevent a too-rapid decrease in the serum osmolality, which could lead to cerebral edema. Potassium is added to the fluids when it is established that there is adequate urine output. Glucose is added to the solution generally when serum glucose concentration decreases to 300 mg/dL, then usually 5% dextrose with half-normal or normal saline solution is used.

121. Why is insulin initially given by continuous infusion in DKA?

An **insulin infusion** is recommended initially so that careful attention can be paid to the rate of correction of **hyperglycemia**. An infusion, started at a level of 0.05–0.1 U/kg/hr of regular insulin, allows the nurse to titrate the level to achieve the desired glucose level. Hyperglycemia must be corrected slowly (≤ 10% decrease every hour). Even after glucose is added to the infusions, it is important to continue the insulin infusion to maintain the serum glucose to prevent a too-rapid decrease in serum osmolality.

122. What is the major complication of DKA?

Cerebral edema. Clinically, cerebral edema occurs in children with DKA after institution of therapy as the clinical and laboratory findings are improving. Although the exact cause is unknown, it is thought that the rapid fall in blood glucose from a hyperosmolar state and a rapid administration of intravenous fluids may contribute to its development.

123. List signs and symptoms of cerebral edema the nurse should assess for.

Headache	Decreased pupil reactivity
Altered level of consciousness	Hypertension
Bradycardia	Abnormal respiratory patterns

124. What agent is used for treatment of ICP in DKA?

Mannitol.

125. You are caring for a 2-year-old patient 2 days after an astrocytoma resection. You notice that her urine output has been 10 mL/kg for the last 2 hours. What do you suspect that the patient is developing?

Neurogenic diabetes insipidus. Diabetes insipidus is a disorder that results in excessive thirst and urination, involving a hormone deficiency in the pituitary gland located at the base of the brain. The hormone that is deficient is **antidiuretic hormone (ADH)**. ADH is responsible for telling the kidneys to hold onto water. When there is a deficiency of this hormone, excess water is excreted, and the patient becomes dehydrated.

126. List causes of diabetes insipidus.

- Tumor of the pituitary gland
- Head injury
- Brain tumors
- Infections such as meningitis and encephalitis
- Hemorrhage in the pituitary gland or surrounding structures
- Aneurysm

127. What form of diabetes insipidus originates in the kidney?

Nephrogenic diabetes insipidus.

128. How is diabetes insipidus treated?

Treatment focuses on **fluid management** and administration of **desmopressin acetate** (DDAVP). The patient often is dehydrated and must be rehydrated to **euvolemia**. Patients often have significant hypernatremia and require careful administration of intravenous fluids with high enough tonicity to avoid acute decreases in serum osmolality. Acute changes in osmolality can lead to significant shifts of fluid into brain cells and potentiate cerebral edema. After euvolemia is obtained, fluid management often starts with insensible output (400–600 mL/m^2/day), plus urine output replacement millimeter for millimeter. Replacing urine output avoids further dehydration resulting from high urinary fluid losses. DDAVP is a synthetic analog of arginine vasopressin, which possesses antidiuretic activity. It increases absorption of water in the kidney by increasing permeability of cells in the collecting ducts. Serum sodium must be monitored closely during treatment. After initiation of DDAVP, fluid management often can be adjusted. In situations of postoperative tumors, meningitis, encephalitis, and hemorrhage, DI can be transient and abate during the critical care admission.

129. What is the syndrome of inappropriate antidiuretic hormone (SIADH)?
The continued secretion of ADH despite low serum osmolality and expanded extracellular volume. The mechanism of SIADH is not clearly understood, but in many circumstances there is direct involvement with the hypothalamus.

130. What are the common signs of SIADH?

Low serum sodium value	Irritability
Low urine output	Nausea and vomiting
Seizures	Personality change
Normotension with increased extracellular fluid	

131. What are the laboratory findings in SIADH?

Low serum sodium	Less than maximally dilute urine
Low serum chloride	High urine sodium
Serum hypo-osmolality	

132. Which patients in the intensive care unit are at risk for developing SIADH?
Patients who have diseases involving the central nervous system:

Meningitis	Brain tumors
Encephalitis	Head trauma

133. What is the mechanism of action in SIADH in situations with tumor involvement?
The tumor presumably synthesizes and secretes ADH.

134. What other clinical situations are associated with SIADH at a lesser rate of occurrence?

Pneumonia	Perinatal asphyxia
Tuberculosis	Chemotherapeutic agents, such as vincristine and vinblastine
Cystic fibrosis	Positive-pressure ventilation

135. How is SIADH treated?
Management of SIADH consists of **fluid restriction** to insensible fluid replacement ($400 \text{ mL/m}^2/\text{day}$), **replacement of sodium losses**, and consideration of **diuretics**.
   1. Insensible fluid administration provides the patient with fluid replacement of estimated ongoing losses from breathing, moving, and maintaining a normal temperature.
   2. Serum sodium values are low in these patients as a result of fluid overload and dilution. In cases of seizure activity related to hyponatremia, hypertonic saline increases the osmolality and controls the central nervous system manifestations.
   3. Diuretic therapy increases free water losses resulting from volume overload.

RENAL FAILURE

136. Why is administration of potassium chloride dangerous in children with acute renal failure?
Patients with acute renal failure accumulate **potassium** because the kidney is responsible for 85–90% of potassium excretion. The remaining potassium is excreted through the gastrointestinal tract. Patients with acute renal failure, plus rhabdomyolysis, hemolysis, or tissue necrosis, have a large release of intracellular potassium. When a patient has a decrease in potassium excretion coupled with increase in production or in exogenous administration of potassium levels, the serum potassium may reach dangerously high levels. Acidosis also

leads to **hyperkalemia**. For every decrease in pH by 0.1 unit, potassium level is increased by 0.5 mEq/L. Hyperkalemia is life-threatening because of the importance of the intracellular potassium gradient in regulation of the cardiac potential. Hyperkalemia can lead to ventricular fibrillation and death and must be treated aggressively.

137. How does sodium polystyrene sulfonate (Kayexalate) work in reducing a child's serum potassium level?

Kayexalate exchanges potassium for sodium in the intestine. Potassium is excreted primarily in the colon, making it possible to administer Kayexalate orally, via nasogastric tube, or as an enema. Normally the dose is 1 g resin/kg/dose every 4–6 hours.

138. Identify concerns with the use of Kayexalate.
- Kayexalate may cause hypomagnesemia, hypocalcemia, diarrhea, and gastric irritation.
- Care should be taken to ensure the child can maintain a patent airway, or the child should intubated to avoid complications with aspiration of vomit.

THE DYING CHILD

139. How should the nurse answer the dying child who asks about his or her prognosis?

The nurse should never lie about the prognosis. The child's developmental level and age always should be considered when speaking to the child about death.

140. Identify the most important need of dying children.

To have the presence of parents and family members in an ongoing fashion. Parents and family members should be allowed to stay with the child as much as they are able.

141. How can the nurse help parents after the death of their child?
- Parents must be given a private place to grieve for their child.
- Health care professionals should be available for support.
- Listening to the parents' memories of their child and sharing your own can be helpful.
- Parents must be allowed private time to say goodbye to the child after the death.

CONTROVERSY

142. Discuss the use of heparin infusion therapy in DIC.

The intended purpose of heparin therapy is to prevent further activation of the clotting cascade, but the effectiveness of this treatment is questionable. The fibrinogen level is the most valuable test for effectiveness of heparin—it should rise to a normal level in 24–48 hours.

BIBLIOGRAPHY

1. Curley MAQ, Moloney-Harmon P (eds): Critical Care Nursing of Infants and Children, 2nd ed. St. Louis, Mosby, 2001.
2. Fuhrman B, Zimmerman J (eds): Pediatric Critical Care, 2nd ed. St. Louis, Mosby, 1998.
3. Grehn LS: Adverse response to analgesia, sedation and neuromuscular blocking agents in infants and children. AACN Clinical Issues 9:36–48, 1998.
4. Habing C, Bell C: The Pediatric Sedation Resource Manual. Chicago, Children's Memorial Medical Center Handbook, 2000.
5. Levin D, Morris F (eds): Essentials of Pediatric Intensive Care, 2nd ed. New York, Churchill Livingstone, 1997.
6. O'Neill N: Improving ventilation in children using bilevel positive airway pressure. Pediatr Nurs 24:377–382, 1998.
7. Pediatric Advanced Life Support. Dallas, American Heart Association, 1997.
8. Rogers MC, Nichols D (eds): Textbook of Pediatric Intensive Care, 3rd ed. Baltimore, Williams & Wilkins, 1996.

19. NURSING CARE OF THE SURGICAL PATIENT

Beth F. Hallmark, RN, MSN

1. Describe the symptoms of appendicitis.

The signs and symptoms of appendicitis are **abdominal pain**, **tenderness**, and **guarding**. The initial pain may start at the periumbilical area and migrate to the right lower quadrant. McBurney's point is located between the anterosuperior iliac crest and umbilical area; children often describe the pain as most severe in this area. Movement may aggravate the pain.

2. What significant history is associated with appendicitis?

The child may have a history of nausea and vomiting or diarrhea.

3. List assessment data you might find when an appendix ruptures.

- WBC 15,000–20,000/mm^3
- Temperature > 101.5°F (38.33°C)
- Sudden relief of pain, followed later by increased pain
- Progressive abdominal distention
- Signs and symptoms of peritonitis
- Guarding
- Abdomen tight on palpation
- Signs and symptoms of septic process
- Tachycardia
- Increased respirations and shallow breathing
- Chills

4. What is an I&D?

An **incision and drainage** (I&D) is performed when infection or fluid has become trapped. An I&D is done to facilitate healing or obtain a culture. After the skin is cleansed, the practitioner incises the infected area with a knife blade and drains the fluid from the wound. The wound subsequently is dressed or packed.

5. State nursing care of the child after an I&D.

The wound is irrigated and commonly packed with wet-to-dry dressings.

6. The normal saline used to irrigate the wound should be at what temperature before wound care?

Warm.

7. What is short bowel syndrome?

A decrease in the mucosal surface area of the intestine. Short bowel syndrome usually is related to the surgical removal of a large portion of small intestine. The physiologic result is **malabsorption**.

8. List conditions that often are related to surgical removal of the small intestine.

Hirschsprung's disease   Omphalocele
Necrotizing enterocolitis   Other conditions that result in bowel necrosis
Gastroschisis

9. Describe types of venous access devices that are used for total parenteral nutrition and intralipids infusion in children with short bowel syndrome.

Peripherally inserted central catheters (PICC). A PICC most commonly is inserted into the superior vena cava. A PICC is inserted through the antecubital vein and can be inserted under radiologic guidance. These catheters typically are not seen in long-term home use. PICCs are inserted by registered nurses who have had special training.

Tunneled catheter. A tunneled catheter is inserted via the subclavian vein into the superior vena cava and ultimately terminates in the right atrium. The catheters are made with cuffs that encourage adherence of the catheter and ultimately aid in stabilization and prevent or decrease the migration of infectious organisms, decreasing the risk of infection. A tunneled catheter is often a multilumen catheter. The catheters can be identified by the brand names **Broviac** or **Hickman**.

10. When flushing a PICC catheter, what syringe should be used and why?

The Intravenous Nursing Society recommends that a **10-mL syringe** be used because it has less pressure per square inch (psi) than a 5-mL syringe. Decreasing psi decreases the risk of catheter rupture.

11. What is intussusception?

Intussusception occurs when the proximal ileum telescopes (invaginates) into the cecum and distal colon (ileocecal valve). As the ileum telescopes, it carries with it the supportive vasculature and causes circulation to be compromised. The telescoping subsequently can lead to necrosis and eventual perforation if not corrected.

12. List the cardinal clinical symptoms of intussusception.

- The **currant-jelly stool**, a combination of blood and mucus resulting from the edema and obstruction caused by the circulatory compromise
- Abdominal pain with cramping
- Bleeding from the rectum
- Nausea and vomiting
- Abdominal distention

13. How is intussusception corrected?

Under **fluoroscopy**, a catheter is inserted and secured in the rectum (the buttocks are taped together to obtain an occlusive seal). Subsequently, either radiopaque barium under hydrostatic pressure or simple pneumatic pressure fills the colon and persuades the cecum to return to the correct position. If this is unsuccessful, a **surgical reduction** with possible bowel resection is performed.

14. Relate important discharge instructions for the parents of a child who has a reduction of intussusception.

Recurrence is possible.
Signs and symptoms of bowel obstruction:

Nausea and vomiting	Swollen (distended) abdomen
Abdominal pain and cramping	Lethargic

15. What is a meconium ileus?

The meconium essentially obstructs the ileum. The neonate presents with a distended abdomen, vomiting, and failure to pass the meconium.

16. When a neonate is diagnosed with a meconium ileus, what disease process should the practitioner consider?

Cystic fibrosis causes the meconium to be viscous with a decreased water content.

17. Summarize the two most common types of irritable bowel disease.

	ULCERATIVE COLITIS	CROHN'S DISEASE
Types of lesions	Continuous Superficial	Segmental Full wall thickness
Areas of involvement	Colon, rectum	Anywhere from mouth to anus
Signs and symptoms	Mild-to-moderate anorexia Severe diarrhea Mild growth retardation Rectal bleeding Moderate weight loss Abdominal pain less common Fistulas rare	Severe anorexia Moderate diarrhea Significant growth retardation No rectal bleeding Significant weight loss Abdominal pain common Fistulas common
Surgical treatment	Subtotal colectomy Ileostomy J pouch with ileoanal pull- through Surgery curative	Resections may be performed, but disease often recurs
Risk of cancer	Long-term complication; surgical resection often cures disease and eliminates risk of cancer	Not common; however, surgery does not decrease incidence

18. What is a pectus excavatum?
Depression of the lower portion of the sternum.

19. What should the nurse take into consideration when caring for a patient with a possible pectus excavatum?
If severe, a pectus excavatum may affect the respiratory or cardiac systems. A pectus excavatum can have psychological effects. As the child enters adolescence and body image becomes important, he or she likely will seek a surgical repair.

20. Define extracorporeal membrane oxygenation (ECMO).
ECMO is used to rest the lungs to provide healing time, using cardiopulmonary bypass. The ECMO device is cannulated through the arterial or venous system and oxygenates the body while resting the lungs.

21. When is ECMO indicated?
Lipoid aspiration   Near-drowning
Cardiac surgery   Acute respiratory failure

22. What is a tracheoesophageal fistula (TEF)?
A congenital birth defect in which the trachea and esophagus are connected via a fistula.

23. List signs and symptoms in a neonate with a TEF.
Excessive frothy saliva
Difficulty handling secretions
Gagging on feedings that return to the nose or mouth

24. Describe the nurse's role in caring for the infant with a TEF.
The nurse should be alert to episodes of cyanosis and immediately clear the airway. Preserving lung function and preventing injury to the respiratory tract are the primary goals of

the nurse. Because surgical repair may not be immediate, the neonate will require continuous monitoring. An orogastric tube is passed and connected to suction to provide for removal of saliva and secretions.

25. What is esophageal atresia?

The absence of the terminal portion of the esophagus. The esophagus ends in a blind pouch. Esophageal atresia often is associated with TEF.

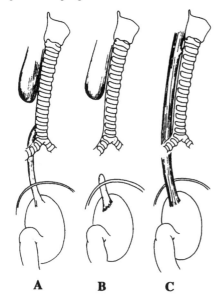

Esophageal atresia. *A,* The most common form of esophageal atresia (85%) consists of a dilated proximal esophageal pouch and a connection of the distal esophagus to the carina of the trachea. *B,* Pure esophageal atresia. *C,* Fistula of the H-type without atresia. (From Coran AG (ed): Surgery of the Neonate. Boston, Little, Brown, 1978, p 46, with permission.)

A   B   C

26. Describe the characteristics often found in necrotizing enterocolitis (NEC).

NEC is associated with **low–birth-weight infants**. There is an increased risk in infants weighing < 1500 g. NEC is related to several factors that often are more common in the premature neonate. The presence of bacteria in the lumen of the bowel, the introduction of a substrate with formula, and an ischemic event all contribute to NEC.

27. Summarize assessment of the infant with NEC.

Abdominal assessment:
Abdominal circumference
Auscultate for bowel sounds
Assess for distention—abdomen may appear shiny
Hemoccult stool
Hemoccult emesis
Intake and output:
Vomiting (may be bile stained)
Urine output
Monitor respiratory status for apnea
Monitor for signs and symptoms of sepsis:
Temperature instability (frequently hypothermic)
Decreased heart rate
Hypotension
Lethargy
The nurse should recognize which infants are at **high risk** for developing NEC and maintain the assessment of these infants.

28. What medical condition sometimes is associated with rectal prolapse and why?

Cystic fibrosis can contribute to rectal prolapse. The malfunctioning (constipation, diarrhea, malabsorption, chronic distention, large bulky fatty stools, and cramping) within the bowel of a child with cystic fibrosis contributes to the prolapse.

29. What is an imperforate anus?

The absence of the terminal anus or rectum or both. Imperforate anus is classified according to the defect's location. Low defects cross or intersect the puborectalis muscle, whereas high defects terminate above this important landmark. Imperforate anus can range from an absent rectum and anus to a rectovaginal fistula.

30. How is imperforate anus diagnosed?

- Imperforate anus can be discovered as the nurse completes the neonatal admission assessment. The normal anal opening would not be observed.
- The location of an imperforate anus cannot be noted until an ultrasound is performed.
- Stool should be noted exiting from the rectum in the event a rectovaginal fistula has formed; otherwise the defect could go undiagnosed at birth.

31. True or false? Gastroschisis is an abdominal wall defect that occurs when the bowel herniates through the umbilical ring and is covered by the peritoneal sac.

False. Gastroschisis is an abdominal wall defect, but the bowel herniates to the right of the umbilicus, and the bowel is exposed with no covering. Omphalocele is an abdominal wall defect that occurs when the bowel herniates through the umbilical ring and is covered by the peritoneal sac.

32. What is the first nursing care priority in the stable newborn with an abdominal wall defect?

Covering the defect and sterile saline gauze. After covering the defect with sterile saline-soaked gauze, the gauze is covered in plastic wrap to prevent excessive, insensible losses that occur through evaporation and to prevent radiant heat loss.

33. Compare nursing care priorities for neonates with omphalocele versus neonates with gastroschisis.

Because the **peritoneal sac** covers the bowel in a neonate with **omphalocele**, the neonate is less susceptible to infection and bowel rupture than the neonate with **gastroschisis**. Gastroschisis and omphalocele increase the risk for fluid and electrolyte imbalance, and intravenous fluids should be started expediently in both cases, and the neonate should be monitored closely for signs and symptoms of dehydration.

34. What is congenital diaphragmatic hernia (CDH)?

A diaphragmatic hernia is documented in approximately 1 in 2000–4000 births. The defect occurs between the 8th and 10th weeks of gestation. A CDH results when there is a defect in the diaphragm, allowing bowel to herniate into the thoracic area, compromising lung development and subsequent respiratory function. A complication is related to the herniation of the liver into the thorax, further compromising lung growth and function.

35. How is a CDH diagnosed?

By **ultrasound**. A diagnosis at 25 weeks' gestation can improve outcomes significantly.

36. What are the three main characteristics that ultrasound reveals?

1. Polyhydramnios
2. Mediastinal shift
3. Stomach not identifiable as evidenced by the **bubble**

37. What are the common treatment options after prenatal diagnosis of CDH?
• Surgery performed immediately after delivery
• Surgery performed after the infant shows stabilization of cardiopulmonary function
• ECMO to allow for pulmonary respite
• Fetal surgery, which allows for the lungs to reach their full development

38. Give two examples of protein hydrosylate formulas.
Nutramigen
Pregestimil

39. Why are protein hydrosylate formulas frequently used in the pediatric surgery patient?
The protein found in these formulas is the **casein hydrosylate protein**, which is digested easily. Neonates who have had any type of intestinal surgery or injury can benefit from the use of elemental formulas. The casein protein allows the bowel to digest the protein with less difficulty. Pregestimil consists of a **predigested** protein, and the kilocalories that come from fat are derived from medium-chain triglyceride oil. Medium-chain triglyceride oil is digested more easily than the fats present in traditional formulas. Pregestimil also contains no sucrose or lactose; the carbohydrates are added via cornstarch. All of these variations allow Pregestimil and other protein hydrosylate formulas to be digested more easily.

40. What is a gastrostomy tube?
A feeding tube that allows for feedings to be administered directly into the stomach. Gastrostomy tubes exit the stomach through the anterior wall and terminate on the abdominal wall.

41. What is the most common type of gastrostomy tube?
The **Stamm gastrostomy** tube is the most common type placed in pediatric patients. It is placed surgically through the incision in the stomach via abdominal wall, and the stomach is attached surgically to the peritoneal wall. This is a permanent attachment and helps prevent leakage of formula into the peritoneal cavity.

42. How is a Stamm gastrostomy placed?
The Stamm gastrostomy uses a mushroom-shaped (Pessar) catheter or a Foley catheter that can be converted to a skin level device 4–6 weeks postoperatively.

43. Name the two most common types of skin level devices.
The Bard Button (Bard Endoscopic Technologies, Billerica, MA) and the Mic-KEY device (Medical Innovations Corp., Santa Clara, CA).

44. Why is the skin level device is preferred?
• The skin level device enables the child and or parents to hide the tube under clothing.
• The tubing is not attached permanently. decreasing the likelihood of accidental removal by the child.
• There is no reason to dress the device when a tract has formed and skin is healthy.

45. How does a percutaneous endoscopic gastrostomy tube differ from a Stamm gastrostomy tube?
A percutaneous endoscopic gastrostomy tube is placed endoscopically and is not a long-term solution to feeding disorders.

46. Name five reasons gastrostomy tubes are placed.
1. To increase kilocalories in a child with cystic fibrosis who has wasting related to malabsorption.

2. To increase kilocalories in a child with cancer to assist in nutritional requirements.

3. To provide total or partial nutrition in a child or infant with gastroesophageal reflux.

4. To provide supplemental or total kilocalorie intake in the neurologically delayed child.

5. To allow for continuous administration of feedings to an infant or child with microgastria or feeding intolerance.

47. What is a Nissen fundoplication?

The surgical wrapping of the fundus of the stomach 360° around the terminal esophagus to prevent gastroesophageal reflux (GER). A Nissen fundoplication helps control GER associated with negative sequelae such as aspiration pneumonia.

48. How is a child evaluated for GER before a gastrostomy tube placement?

An upper gastrointestinal study under fluoroscopy.

49. Why is the gastrostomy tube catheter vented (via an elevated syringe) postoperatively?

The catheter is open to gravity or vented until peristalsis returns to the bowel. This decompresses the stomach similar to a nasogastric tube after gastrointestinal surgery.

50. How do the rationales for bolus and continuous feedings differ?

- Continuous feedings are used to introduce formula slowly back into the stomach and gastrointestinal tract.
- Frequently, continuous feedings are started postoperatively to allow the stomach and gastrointestinal tract to become tolerant of small volumes until full function returns to the gastrointestinal tract.
- A continuous feeding would be used in the infant or child who has severe GER and cannot tolerate the volume a bolus delivers (as evidence by retching and gagging during feeds).
- Continuous feeds optimally are given via a feeding pump.
- Bolus feedings are given in a certain volume over several minutes.
- Bolus feedings often are more convenient for the family because the feeding is done, then the tube is clamped.

51. Should bolus feedings be given by pushing a plunger into a syringe?

No, bolus feedings are tolerated best if allowed to infuse via gravity.

52. Discuss ways to enable the patient to tolerate bolus feedings more easily.

- Bolus feedings are tolerated more easily if they are given with the developmental age and neurologic condition of the child considered.
- The neurologically devastated child needs to get his or her feedings over a longer period than the child who is receiving gastrostomy tube feedings to increase kilocalories.
- Frequently neurologically devastated children cannot tolerate bolus feeds and must be monitored closely because of their risk for aspiration and reflux.
- Placing the child in a head-up position during feeds and for 30 minutes after feeds can minimize the risk for reflux-related complications.

53. What are the advantages and disadvantages of performing a Nissen fundoplication?

The advantage is weight gain. The disadvantages include (1) asthma and (2) frequent respiratory infections with respiratory difficulty (e.g., wheezing, rales).

54. Define Hirschsprung's disease.

The congenital absence of parasympathetic ganglion cells. The absence of these cells results in atypical peristalsis.

55. What early sign may alert the nurse that a neonate might have Hirschsprung's disease?

Failure of the meconium to pass.

56. List signs and symptoms of Hirschsprung's disease in the infant or child.

History of constipation	Explosive passage of stool gas on rectal examination
Abdominal distention	Ribbon shape of the stool
Bilious emesis	

57. When projectile vomiting is reported in a 4-week-old male firstborn infant, the practitioner would investigate further the possibility of which obstructive disorder?

Pyloric stenosis, also called **hypertrophic pyloric stenosis**, a condition in which the pyloric muscle becomes increasingly thickened and results in an obstruction at the pylorus.

58. Describe the appearance of the emesis of an infant with pyloric stenosis.

Formula can be seen in the emesis or streaks of blood related to esophageal irritation. Bile is not found because the location of the obstruction is proximal to the inlet to the duodenum (small intestine).

59. What acid-base disturbance would you suspect in an infant with pyloric stenosis, a 2-day history of projectile vomiting, and the following laboratory values: sodium, 134 mEq/L; potassium, 4.5 mEq/L; chloride, 110 mEq/L; pH, 7.29; and bicarbonate, 20 mEq/L?

Metabolic acidosis.

60. What condition has led to metabolic acidosis?

The excessive loss of **fluid and electrolytes** related to the 2-day history of emesis and inability to retain oral fluids.

61. Prioritize and provide the rationale for interventions for a 3-week-old infant admitted with a diagnosis of rule-out pyloric stenosis.

PRIORITY	INTERVENTION	RATIONALE
1	Weight infant	The infant must be weighed first for the intravenous fluids to be calculated and to help determine the degree of dehydration present.
2	Intravenous fluids	After the infant in weighed, fluids can be infused.
3	Administer potassium	Any necessary potassium replacement that may be needed for depletion that has occurred can be infused next.
4	Immunization history	The immunization history is an important piece of the infant's history after he or she is stabilized.

62. True or false? Breast milk is considered a clear liquid postoperatively.

True. Most surgeons and anesthesiologists consider breast milk a clear liquid related to its low osmolality.

63. Name three pain scales that commonly are used with children.

SCALE	AGE (YR)
FACES pain rating scale	≥ 3
Numeric scale	Typically ≥ 5
Oucher scale	≥ 3

64. Describe the cognitive and psychosocial development of the infant.

The infant is in Erikson's stage of trust versus mistrust and Piaget's sensorimotor stage. Some typical behaviors of the infant are:

Consumption of food and formula	Cause and effect
Egocentric	Curious
Grasping	Object permanence
Easily frustrated	

65. List some preoperative preparation interventions that support the infant's psychosocial and cognitive development.

- Eye contact
- Soft soothing words
- Parent or primary caregiver present
- Meet physical needs as much as possible (i.e., pick up when crying, pacifier if NPO, feed as soon as possible)

66. Describe the cognitive and psychosocial development of the toddler.

The toddler is in Erikson's stage of autonomy versus shame and doubt and Piaget's preoperational stage. Some typical behaviors of the toddler are:

Negativism	Egocentric
Ritualism	Concrete thinking
Potty-training	Transductive thinking

67. List some preoperative preparation interventions that support the toddler's psychosocial and cognitive development.

Honesty	Music
Parental presence	Realistic choices
Transitional object	Use of toys and play in preparation
Premedication	

68. List some typical behaviors of the preschool child that should be considered in preoperative preparation.

Magical thinking	Play important
Self-blame	Concrete thinking
Fear of body mutilation	Animism
Inability to understand time	

69. How long before a procedure should you prepare a preschool child?

Preoperative preparation for a child aged 2–5 years should not be done more than a day in advance. Depending on their specific age, young children do not have an understanding of time, and preparing them too far in advance causes increased anxiety.

70. What preoperative preparation interventions support the preschooler's psychosocial and cognitive development?

- Puppets
- Covering wounds and incisions with bandages
- Honesty
- Picture books with verbal explanation
- Parental presence
- Premedication
- Explanations of time by using events they understand
- Using toys to distract
- Music

- Telling child it is okay to be scared
- Letting child touch equipment
- Explaining sounds and sights

71. How is preoperative preparation influenced by the cognitive and psychosocial development of the school-age child?

The school-age child is in Erikson's stage of industry versus inferiority and Piaget's preoperational and concrete and formal operations stages. Some typical behavior characteristics of the school-age child are:

Achievement	Egocentric period ends	Cooperation
Completing tasks	Reversibility	Friends important
Collections	Reciprocity	School important

72. What preoperative preparation interventions support the school-age child's psychosocial and cognitive development?

Pictures with explanation	Give permission to be scared
Parents	Distract with music
Friends	Explain sounds and sights
Encourage child to verbalize fears	Privacy

73. Describe how preoperative preparation can be influenced by the cognitive and psychosocial development of the adolescent.

The adolescent is in Erikson's stage of identity versus role confusion and Piaget's formal operations stage. Some typical behaviors of the adolescent are:

Abstract thought	Intellect important
Peers important	Self-centered
Conformity	Invincible

74. What preoperative preparation interventions support the adolescent's psychosocial and cognitive development?

- Peers important—introduce teen to peer with same procedure
- Pictures and verbal and written instructions
- Privacy
- Allow teen to express feelings and fears

75. Name five tasks the circulating nurse performs.

1. Verifies the child's name and identity.
2. Confirms the expected procedure with the child's parents.
3. Clarifies any concerns the family might have, either directly or through the surgeon or anesthesiologist.
4. Reviews all paper work to verify inclusion of order and consent, laboratory test results, radiographs, history and physical examination results.
5. Performs a brief assessment of the child to determine cognitive ability and psychosocial behaviors.

76. Why are children at greater risk for temperature instability than adults during surgery?

Children have a much greater surface body area than adults.

77. Through what two mechanisms does temperature decrease rapidly in children during operative procedures?

1. Evaporative and insensible losses—through visceral exposure intraoperatively.
2. Convective losses—when the child is exposed to large volumes of fluid on the skin and fluids pool under the child.

78. Temperature instability can result in what operative complication?

When the child becomes hypothermic, **hypoxia** can result, increasing oxygen consumption and subsequently putting the child at risk for oxygen deprivation.

79. What additional factors should be monitored carefully during the surgical procedure?
- Urine output
- Skin integrity
- Laboratory values as ordered to monitor problems related to blood loss

80. Identify three nursing diagnoses that the nurse should document in the plan of care for a child undergoing a routine surgical procedure.

1. Alteration in skin integrity related to surgical incision, positioning in the operating room, and immobility.
2. Alteration in fluid and electrolyte balance.
3. Alteration in gas exchange related to anesthesia.

81. What are the three most important nursing concerns when caring for a pediatric patient during a surgical procedure?

1. Temperature regulation
2. Fluid and electrolyte imbalance
3. Positioning and skin integrity

82. When monitoring the urine output of a postoperative child, how much urine should the postanesthesia care unit nurse expect?

The urine output should be 1 mL/kg/hr for children who have no underlying problem with fluid overload. If a child is on fluid restrictions or has a high risk for overload problems, the acceptable range is 0.5–1.0 mL/kg/h.

83. What signs and symptoms might the nurse observe that indicate peristalsis has returned after intestinal surgery?
- The child should begin slowly to have bowel sounds that the nurse will be able to auscultate.
- The child should pass flatulence.
- The child may complain of hunger.
- The child may have decreased complaints of nausea.
- The nasogastric tube drainage usually decreases.

84. How can consistency of measurement be ensured among nurses as they assess abdominal circumference on pediatric surgical patients?

By placing the tape slightly above the umbilicus and marking lightly on the skin. Other nurses can use these markings to place the tape for subsequent measurements.

85. What discharge instructions should be given to the family of a child who has undergone a hernia repair?
- Call physician for fever > 101.5°F (38.3°C)
- Do not let child ride straddle toys, such as a tricycle, until approved by the physician.
- Keep the incision clean and dry.
- Call physician if redness, drainage, or swelling occurs at incision.
- Call physician if pain is not relieved by acetaminophen.

BIBLIOGRAPHY

1. Busen NH: Perioperative preparation of the adolescent surgical patient. AORN J 73:335, 337–338, 2001.
2. Carpenter KH: Developing a pediatric/parent hospital preparation program. AORN J 65:1042–1046, 1998.
3. Ellsworth P, Cendron M, Ritland D, McCullough M: Hypospadias repair in the 1990s. AORN J 69:148–161, 1999.
4. George C, Hammes M, Schwarz D: Laparoscopic Swenson pullthrough procedure for congenital megacolon. AORN J 62:727–736, 1995.
5. Glick PL, Pearl RH, Irish MS, Caty MG (eds): Pediatric Surgery Secrets. Philadelphia, Hanley & Belfus, 2001.
6. Wise BV, McKenna C, Garvin G, Harmon BJ (eds): Nursing of the General Pediatric Surgery Patient. Gaithersburg, MD, Aspen, 2000.
7. Wong DL, Hockenberry-Eaton M, Wilson D, et al: Whaley and Wong's Nursing Care of Infants and Children, 6th ed. St. Louis, Mosby, 1999.

20. ISSUES IN SCHOOL HEALTH

Elaine M. Gustafson, MSN, APRN, CS, PNP

1. Why is school health important?

Currently, there are approximately 100,000 schools in the United States, and 45 million children attend these schools. Schools have the potential to deliver health education and services to almost every child in the United States.

2. Name the three traditional components of a school health program.
1. Health instruction
2. Health services
3. Environmental health

3. What are the basic tenets of school health throughout most of the 20th century?
- Classroom-based health education and physical education were the two most important components of school health.
- Private medicine was solely responsible for all medical treatment.
- School health services included emergency care and first aid, keeping records of compliance with state-mandated requirements, and provision of periodic health assessments.
- School health services were defined mainly by the school nurse program.

4. List some current and future school health issues.
- Provision of integrated services by an interdisciplinary team
- Redefinition of the partnership between school nursing and school-based health centers
- Health education with a consumer health and self-care emphasis
- Increased parental involvement in school health issues
- Improved funding of school health services

5. Where did school nursing originate?

In France, when public health services were extended into the schools in 1837. A royal ordinance mandated health supervision of schoolchildren and enforcement of sanitary conditions by school authorities.

6. Where were the first school health services in the United States?

Boston, Massachusetts, in 1894.

7. What was included in the first school health services?

Medical inspection of children for the purpose of exclusion for communicable disease. There was no mechanism for follow-up of these children.

8. Who was responsible for the founding of school nursing in the United States?

Lillian Wald. Early public health work and school nursing in England inspired her.

9. When and where did school nursing begin in the United States?

In 1900 in New York City.

10. Who was the first school nurse?

Lina Rogers Struthers.

11. What was the Henry Street Settlement?
The first nurses' settlement in the United States. It was founded by Lillian Wald and Mary Brewster and was located in New York City's worst slum. Its purpose was to influence the inhabitants by the example of the nurses and by teaching.

12. What are the key components of the school nurse role?
Assessment
Screening
Education
Consultaion

13. What are some of the key issues facing school nursing in the 21st century?
- Increased need for school health services and for the education of school staff
- Necessity for improved physical assessment skills
- Familiarity with high-technology equipment for children with special needs
- Ability to care for students with rare health conditions (e.g., organ transplants, artificial limbs or organs)
- Administration of growing number of psychotropic medications
- Increased number of children with chronic, terminal, and mental illnesses
- Large student-to-nurse ratio

14. Identify some of the political issues and challenges facing school nursing.
- Conflicting goals resulting from dual allegiance to school and health community
- Lack of clear understanding of school nurse role by community
- Necessity to perform non-nursing tasks
- Substandard salaries

15. When were school-based health centers developed?
In the 1970s, the Robert Wood Johnson Foundation funded several demonstration projects leading to the development of school-based health centers.

16. Which health concerns prompted the development of school-based health centers?
- Teenage violence
- Suicide
- Substance abuse
- Pregnancy
- Human immunodeficiency virus (HIV) and acquired immunodeficiency syndrome (AIDS)
- Sexually transmitted diseases

17. What professionals should be included as part of a full-service school-based health center?

Nurse-practitioner	Social worker
Physician consultant	Receptionist

18. What other professionals also may be a part of the team?

Dentist	HIV/AIDS educator
Health educator	Outreach worker

19. Approximately how many school-based health centers are currently in U.S. schools?
> 1300.

20. What populations do school-based health centers serve?
Children in urban and rural areas in elementary, middle, and high schools.

21. Describe the relationship school nursing has with school-based health centers.

School nurses and school-based health center staff act collaboratively to enhance the health and well-being of all schoolchildren. The school nurse is on the front lines making assessments and referring children who may need further assessment and treatment for physical and mental health concerns. A close, collegial relationship between the school nurse and the school-based health center is essential to the efficient running of health services in schools.

22. What are some of the challenges facing school-based health centers?
- Finding new and innovative sources for funding, which are crucial to the continuation of existing school-based health centers and to the development of new centers
- Improved billing and payment schemes
- Development of mechanisms with which to collaborate with primary care providers and others in light of confidentiality mandates

23. What is coordinated school-based health care?

Coordinated school health care is a dynamic partnership between all health personnel in the school, the faculty and administration, and the parents.

24. What are the components of coordinated school-based health care?

Parent and community involvement	Health services
Health promotion for staff	Nutrition services
Health education	Counseling, psychological, and social services
Physical education	Healthy school environment

25. Accomplishing which developmental tasks may facilitate school entry for the young child?
- Positive experience with separation from parents
- Ability to share and take turns as a result of previous interaction with other children
- Ability to perform basic self-care
- Willingness to follow directions
- Development of language skills

26. What could repeated visits to the school nurse signify?
- Anxiety about chronic conditions
- Avoidance of academic problems
- Unresolved physical ailments (e.g., headache, abdominal pain)
- Peer avoidance because of bullying
- School or family issues causing anxiety and inability to cope
- Adjustment problems (e.g., new students, returning students)

27. What roles does the school nurse play in facilitating the child's adjustment to school?
- **Support** and reassurance to the child and parent
- **Liaison** with faculty, administration, and family in facilitation of child's adjustment to school
- **Consultant** to teachers and administrators regarding child's special needs
- **Liaison** with health care providers in support of child's needs
- **Referral** to physical, dental, and mental health care providers when appropriate
- Health **educator** for students, teachers, and administrators regarding specific health concerns

28. List the vaccine-preventable diseases in the school-age child.

Haemophilus influenzae B	Diphtheria	Pertussis
Measles, mumps, and rubella	Tetanus	Hepatitis B
Polio		

29. What are the most common respiratory illnesses spread via fluid from the eyes, nose, mouth, and lungs?

Viral illnesses (colds, influenza)
Group A streptococcal infections
Chickenpox
Fifth disease (erythema infectiosum)
Roseola (especially in the preschool population)
Meningococcal illness
Tuberculosis

30. What is the standard exclusion policy for children with a positive streptococcal culture?

Children should be excluded from school until they have been treated with an antibiotic for 24 hours.

31. Should students with fifth disease be excluded from school?

Possibly. There have been rare reports of miscarriages and stillbirths in women who have contracted fifth disease during pregnancy. This may be of concern to pregnant teachers with students who suffer from fifth disease.

32. What group of students is at highest risk to develop meningococcal disease?

College students living in close proximity in a dormitory setting.

33. What can be done to prevent the spread of infection?

Parents should be alerted to the risk so that they can decide whether to have their child immunized.

34. Which common skin and superficial infections are spread through direct contact?

Impetigo   Scabies
Ringworm (tinea corporis)   Pediculosis (head lice)
Conjunctivitis

35. Which of the above conditions requires immediate treatment?

Pediculosis. Students found to have any of the other conditions usually may complete the school day, then seek treatment or be treated in a school-based health center.

36. Do students with HIV/AIDS pose any risk to their classmates?

No. Students pose no risk of transmission of HIV infection through casual contact that typically occurs at school.

37. Is there any requirement to disclose a diagnosis of HIV/AIDS to school personnel?

No.

38. How prevalent is chronic illness in children?

Some type of chronic condition affects approximately 10–15% of children between the ages of 1 and 19.

39. What percentage of children is afflicted with a severe chronic illness?

1–2%, of which approximately 5% are limited in activities of daily living.

40. Identify some of the potential effects of a chronic illness on a child in school.

• Prolonged absences leading to underachievement
• Limited alertness and stamina as a result of chronic condition or medication effects
• Psychological maladjustment

41. Summarize the federal laws enacted to guarantee children with disabilities access to free and appropriate education.

YEAR	LEGISLATION	PROVISIONS
1973	Section 504 of the Rehabili-tation Act	Prohibits discrimination within federal and federally assisted programs and provides children with chronic and disabling conditions appropriate modification within the school system
1975	Public Law 94-142—Educa-tion for All Handicapped Children Act	Provides that all children have a right to free and appropriate public education in the least restrictive environment. Public schools are required to provide services to correct learning problems
1986	Public Law 99-457	Requires early intervention for children at risk for medical or developmental problems from birth to age 3. Law includes financial assistance in carrying aout the requirements
1990	PL 94-142 (renamed Individuals with Disabilities Education Act [IDEA])	
1997	Amendments to IDEA	Amendments expanded the use of the Individualized Education Program (IEP). The IEP is a written legal document, created by a multidisciplinary team, including parentes, regular education teacher, special education teacher, a representative of the school district, the student, if appropriate, and "other individuals who have special knowledge of the child's disability and needs." The IEP describes the special education and related services to be provided to the student. Amendments also offered financial assistance to carry out the requirements

42. What concerns continue to exist despite the Right of Education laws?
- State and local funding is inadequate for the numbers of children identified with chronic conditions.
- Stricter criteria for special education and associated stigma with labeling have led to placement of children with complex needs in the regular classroom without appropriate support.
- Allocation of resources and funding is geared toward children with severe medical needs versus children needing mental health services.
- Teachers receive little education about children with chronic conditions and psychosocial needs.

43. What condition must be met for a child with a chronic condition to be eligible for special education services?
The child's disability must be shown to have an impact on education performance.

44. State two objectives that relate to physical activity and the school in the *Healthy People 2010* objectives.
1. The proportion of children and adolescents who participate in daily physical activity will increase by 50%.
2. School physical education class time will increase by 50%.

45. What should be the underlying theme in a physical education curriculum?
Health-related fitness that students can apply to their own lifestyle.

46. What are the characteristics of a physically educated person as defined by the National Association for Sport and Physical Education?
- Has necessary skills to perform a variety of physical activities
- Achieves and maintains physical fitness
- Knows the implications and benefits of physical activity
- Values physical activity and its contribution to a healthy lifestyle

47. How many children suffer injuries associated with playground equipment?
> 200,000/yr.

48. What is the most frequent type of injury?
A fall from playground equipment onto the ground.

49. What steps can be taken to prevent playground accidents at school?
- Training of teachers, aides, and volunteers in supervision of children on the playground
- Regular safety checks by trained personnel of playground equipment
- Periodic addition of ground cover to playground surface to ensure that there is at least 12 inches of wood chips, mulch, sand, or pea gravel
- Check that surfacing extends at least 6 feet in all directions from playground equipment
- Playground equipment > 30 inches high should be placed 9 feet apart
- Check for sharp points and tripping hazards
- Playground rules developed by students and teachers and posted where they can be viewed easily

50. Define sick building syndrome.
A **sick building**, also known as a **tight building**, is usually an energy-efficient structure that limits the amount of fresh air entering the building. This leads to the containment and concentration of indoor air pollutants.

51. List some health complaints of individuals who suffer the effects of sick building syndrome.

Eye irritation	Chest tightness	Dizziness
Sinus congestion	Sneezing	Dermatitis
Headache	Nausea	Difficulty wearing contact lenses
Fatigue		

52. Which indoor air pollutants can cause these symptoms?

Carbon monoxide	Ozone
Carbon dioxide	Tobacco smoke
Nitrogen oxide	Microorganisms, such as mold spores, fungi, bacteria, viruses
Radon	Pesticides
Asbestos	

53. What can the school nurse do in the prevention and remediation of sick building syndrome?
Through education, nurses can increase their awareness of environmental hazards in the school. Nurses in turn can educate the community through public education forums and individually by inquiring about potential causes of symptoms. Nurses can encourage advocacy in support of indoor air quality legislation.

54. Why is the use of pesticides of particular concern in schools?
Children are highly susceptible to health damage from many pesticides. Nearly 100 pesticides studied by the Environmental Protection Agency may cause cancer in humans. Children

may be more susceptible because cells are reproducing rapidly as they grow. Pregnant women also should avoid exposure to pesticides because they may pose a risk to the developing fetus.

55. What can be done to reduce the exposure of children to pesticides?
- School personnel should be educated about the use of pesticides, including personnel responsible for maintenance of athletic fields.
- Parents and guardians and school personnel should be notified of the school's pest control policy and should be notified before pesticides are used at school.
- Only trained and certified applicators should spray pesticides on school grounds.
- Data regarding each pesticide application should be kept on file in the school nurse's office.
- Warning labels should be posted around the treated areas of the school.
- Pesticides should not be used while school is in session.
- Schools should never use pesticides for purely aesthetic reasons, such as to keep playing fields looking well.

56. What is bullying?
A form of abuse by peers.

57. List characteristics of bullying.
- Aggressive behavior with intention to do harm
- Repeated incidents over time
- Occurs in interpersonal relationships based on an imbalance of power
- Occurs without apparent provocation

58. Give some examples of bullying behaviors.

Spreading rumors	Anonymous phone calls
Exclusion from groups	Extortion or stealing
Slandering	Threats and intimidation
Name calling and putdowns	Hitting, teasing, hazing

59. How prevalent is bullying in the United States?
Approximately 10% of children experience extreme victimization by bullying.

60. What causes bullying?
Bullying is the result of a dynamic interaction between the individual and his or her social ecology—family, peers, school, and community.

61. Name two common myths about bullies.
1. Bullies are insecure beneath the bravado.
2. Bullies have poor self-esteem.

62. What are some of the consequences of being a bully?
- Poor school attendance
- Poor academic performance
- Potential for violence and delinquency, such as vandalism, fighting, theft, and substance abuse
- Aggressive behavior at age 8 with no intervention is predictive of criminality and violent behavior and arrest by age 30

63. Summarize ways to address the problem of bullies in school.
- Raise awareness about the problem of bullying through education of school staff.
- Teach children what to do if they are bullied or see someone bullied.
- Suggest **walk, talk, squawk method**—meaning walk away, speak up to a bully, and tell an adult.

• Involve parents.
• Begin a multilevel, multicomponent bully prevention program that involves students, staff, parents, and community.

64. Why are school nutrition programs important?
• For some children, 50–60% of daily nutrients come from school meals.
• Children at risk for undernutrition also are at risk for poor school performance and physical and cognitive deficits.
• Rates of obesity are increasing among children and adolescents.
• Two thirds of school-age children are enrolled in the National School Lunch Program (NSLP)

65. What is the purpose of the NSLP?
NSLP is a federal program enacted in 1946 to allow schools throughout the United States to provide nutritious, low-cost lunches to children each day. Children meeting eligibility criteria may receive free or reduced price lunches.

66. Give some examples of NSLP meals.

Main courses	Vegetables	Fruit
Hamburgers	Iceberg lettuce	Apples
Hot dogs	Raw carrots	Canned peaches
Pizza with meat	Raw tomatoes	Canned pears
Peanut butter sandwiches	Green salads	Fruit cocktail
	French fries	

Milk is the most commonly served beverage.

67. What are the Centers for Disease Control guidelines for nutrition education?
• Develop a school policy on nutrition.
• Offer nutrition curriculum that is coordinated and sequential.
• Combine nutrition education with food services.
• Involve family and community.
• Include staff training on nutrition.

BIBLIOGRAPHY

1. Addiss S, Alderman N, Brown D, et al: Pest Control Practices in Connecticut Public Schools. North Haven, CT, Environment and Human Health, 1999.
2. Anonymous: Handbook for Public Playground Safety (Pub. No. 325). Washington, DC, U.S. Consumer Product Safety Commission, 2000. Available at http://www.cpsc.gov/kids/kidsafety/buddy.html.
3. Briasco ME: Indoor air pollution: Are employees sick from their work? AAOHN J 38:375–380, 1990.
4. Friedrich MJ: 25 Years of school-based health centers. JAMA 281:781–782, 1999.
5. Glew G, Rivara F, Feudtner C: Bullying: Children hurting children. Pediatr Rev 21:183–189, 2000.
6. Goodman L, Sheetz A (eds): The Comprehensive School Health Manual. Boston, Massachusetts Department of Public Health Bureau of Family and Community Health School Health Unit, 1995.
7. Juszczak L, Fisher M: Health care in schools. Adolesc Med State Art Rev 7:163–317, 1996.
8. Olweus D, Limber S: Blueprints for violence prevention. Boulder, CO, Center for the Study and Prevention of Violence, 2000. Available at http://www.colorado.edu/cspv/blueprints/model/chapt/BullyExec.htm.
9. Schwab N, Gelfman M (eds): Legal Issues in School Health Services: A Resource for School Administrators, School Attorneys and School Nurses. North Branch, MN, Sunrise River Press, 2001.

INDEX

Entries in **boldface type** indicate complete chapters.